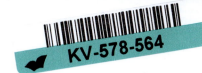

Life

edited by

Mohammad Ali Shomali

Islamic Reference Series:

Vol. 5: Life

Edited by Mohammad Ali Shomali

First published in Great Britain in 2011

ISBN: 978-1-904934-17-2

Published by

Institute of Islamic Studies
Islamic Centre of England
140 Maida Vale, London W9 1QB
Tel: (44) 0207 604 5500; Fax: (44) 0207 604 4898
Email: ic-el@ic-el.com

بسم الله الرحمن الرحيم

In the Name of God,

the Most Gracious, the Most Merciful

Table of Contents

Preface

One of the most important concepts in Islamic thought is the concept of life. A quick review of the Qur'an and the major collections of hadith is enough to confirm the significance of life in all its forms, starting from the life of plants and ending with the life of God Himself. Of course, there is a hierarchy of life and the higher we go within that hierarchy, the more sophisticated and valuable life becomes. In four different verses of the Qur'an, God has been described as "the Living" (*al-Hayy*). In two verses, it has been mentioned immediately after the unity of God (2:255 and 3:2). In another place, it has been mentioned even before the unity of God (40:65). Heaven has been characterised as the Abode of Life (29:64). The entire message of Islam has been introduced as a call towards a new life in addition to the physical life that everyone has been granted by God. The Qur'an says: "O you who have faith! Answer God and the Apostle when he summons you to that which will give you life..." (8:24). This life is the Goodly Life, in which there is no pain or misery; it is full of joy and hope and is available to both men and women: "Whoever acts righteously, [whether] male or female, should he be faithful, We shall revive him with a good life and pay them their reward by the best of what they used to do" (16:97).

Inspired by the Qur'an, Muslim philosophers and mystics believe that, indeed, every creature enjoys some kind of life and, therefore, understanding and love. The Qur'an speaks about the prayer of the birds and their glorification of God, and the glorification of God by the mountains and by Prophet David (a), and the praise and the glorification of God by everything:

We gave its understanding to Solomon, and to each We gave judgement and knowledge. And We disposed the mountains and the birds to glorify [Him] with David, and We have been the Doer [of such things]. (21:79)

Have you not regarded that God is glorified by everyone in the heavens and the earth, and the birds spreading their wings. Each knows his prayer and glorification, and God knows best what they do. (24:41)

This view of the world, in which everything has life and understanding, manifests God, acts as His sign, and has been created by Him for a purpose, bestows an intrinsic value to everything. Animals, plants and even non-living beings are valuable by themselves and not just for what we can gain from them. A Muslim must act as a guardian of the environment and try to improve its conditions. Such understanding of the world leaves no room for destroying nature or even disrespecting animals, plants and natural resources, let alone disregarding human life. According to the Qur'an, "whoever kills a soul, without [its being guilty of] manslaughter or corruption on the earth, is as though he had killed all mankind, and whoever saves a life is as though he had saved all mankind" (5:32). This is quite opposite to the view that life is created by chance and that man can live his life as he wishes and *use* other forms of life as suits his interests. Suicide, abortion, murder, unending wars, the pollution of air, rivers and lakes, and the destruction of forests and farms are a few of the outcomes of this attitude to life.

The people of our age are in need of constant reflection on life in order to better appreciate their physical lives and the lives of others and find their path towards the spiritual life. Believers should feel the presence of God, the Living, who sees them (96:14), and act responsibly in order to make the Goodly Life possible for themselves and for others.

The papers which are included in this volume examine different aspects of the Islamic understanding of life. In addition to divine life, created life, in both its physical and spiritual forms, is discussed. Most of the papers included here have been translated from Farsi or Arabic specifically for this volume and are being published for the first time in English. This will give readers the opportunity to become familiar with a number of contemporary thinkers in the Muslim world and to get acquainted with their scholarship.

The first essay is entitled "Islamic Bioethics: A General Scheme." In this paper, Dr. Mohammad Ali Shomali seeks to provide a general account of life in Islam. In the first part of the article, the value of life and its sacredness are explored, while in the second part, Islamic regulations for safeguarding human life are examined. The maintenance of physical health and the treatment of the sick are singled out as examples which are used to illustrate the necessity of protecting life. With regard to the beginning of human life, stress has been put on family as a stable and legitimate context for producing and raising children. With respect to the end of life, issues such as abortion, euthanasia, suicide and brain death are addressed. This paper includes some of the ideas which were originally presented in conferences in London, Leeds, New York, Minsk and Tehran. It was first published in the *Journal of Medical Ethics and History of Medicine,* 1:1 (2008), by the Tehran University of Medical Sciences and is now published here with a few changes.

The second paper is entitled "God, the Living." In this short paper, Ayatollah Ja'far Subhani examines God's quality of life. Referring to what scientists and philosophers have asserted as the definition of life in its three forms i.e. the vegetative life, the animal life and human life, the author tries to discover what is common to all different forms of life and ends with an explanation of divine life as the most perfect form of life which has no beginning or end. This paper is an excerpt from the first volume of *Al-Ilāhiyyāt* (vols. 1-3) by Ayatollah Ja'far Subhani

(Qum: Imam Sadiq Institute, 2005). This paper has been translated from Arabic into English for this volume by Vahid Mohammadi and Mohammad Javad Shomali.

The third paper is entitled "Human Life." In this paper, Ayatollah Misbah Yazdi considers human life as distinct from vegetative life and animal life. He elucidates the manner in which human beings can achieve light and spiritual life in this world and the Hereafter. This paper was published in *Ma'ārif-e Ja'fari*, Issue 6, March 1966, and has been translated from Farsi into English for this volume by Vahid Mohammadi and Mohammad Javad Shomali.

The fourth paper is entitled "The Fundamentality of the Soul." In this paper, the late Ayatollah Mutahhari analyses the relation between the soul and the body. Exploring the issue of life and the soul from a philosophical perspective, he first criticises the ideas of those who hold that the soul is a property or an effect of matter and then argues that matter lacks life in its nature and that life is a reality on its own with certain features that cannot be found in matter. This paper was published in the *Maktab-e Tashayyu'*, Issue Zero, April 1959, and has been has been translated from Farsi into English for this volume by Vahid Mohammadi and Mohammad Javad Shomali.

The fifth paper is entitled "The Qur'an and Life." In this paper, the late Ayatollah Mutahhari tries to present a Qur'anic account of life. In particular, he tries to explore the relation between human life, the supernatural world and divine life. This paper was published in the *Maktab-e Tashayyu'*, Issue 1, September 1959, and has been translated from Farsi into English for this volume by Vahid Mohammadi and Mohammad Javad Shomali.

The sixth paper is entitled "The Goodly Life from a Qur'anic Perspective." In this paper, Hujjat al-Islam Hamid Mazaheri Seif presents an articulate account of the Goodly Life (*al-Hayāt al-Tayyibah*): its meaning, requirements and outcomes. He also explains the notion of the world-with-God and its relation with the Goodly Life and Divine Guardianship (*wilāyah*). This paper was published in *Ma'rifat*, Issue 109, January 2007, by the Imam Khomeini Education and Research Institute, Qum. It has been translated from Farsi into English for this volume by Vahid Mohammadi and Mohammad Javad Shomali.

The seventh paper is entitled "Respect for Animal Life in Islam." In this paper, Hujjat al-Islam Ali Ahmadi Khah examines the status of animals in Islam. Referring to the Sunnah of Prophet Muhammad (s), the author argues that Islam has a high regard for both the preservation of animal life and the improvement of the conditions of their life. This paper was published in *Tārikh dar A'ineh Pazhuhesh*, Issue 11, Autumn 2006, by the Imam Khomeini Education and Research Institute, Qum. It has been translated from Farsi into English for this volume by Mohammad Javad Shomali.

The eighth and final paper is entitled "Aspects of Environmental Ethics: An Islamic Perspective." In this paper, Dr. Mohammad Ali Shomali refers to the emphasis which is given to nature by the Holy Qur'an and then focuses on the significance of water, earth, plants and animals in the Holy Qur'an and Sunnah. He argues that the environment has an intrinsic value and that, as the vicegerents of God, we have to channel the mercy of God into everything within our reach. This paper was first presented in a conference on "Faiths in Creation" at Heythrop College, University of London on 12th June 2008. It was published in *Faith in Creation* (The Institute Series) by the Heythrop Institute for Religion, Ethics and Public Life, September 2008, and is now published here with a few changes.

I would like to thank everyone who has contributed to this volume and I pray for their success in both their personal and academic lives. I would also like to thank Kawther Rahmani of the U.S. for editing the entire volume and making valuable comments. In addition, I would like to thank Hujjat al-Islam wa'l-

Muslimin Abdulhusein Moezzi, the Director of the Islamic Centre of England, for his support and encouragement. And last, but by no means least, I would like to thank God, the Almighty, for His Guidance and Favour upon us in both past and present.

Mohammad Ali Shomali

March 2011

أُدْخُلُوهَا بِسَلَامٍ آمِنِينَ

ENTER IT IN PEACE AND SECURITY

(46:15)

Islamic Bioethics: A General Scheme

Mohammad Ali Shomali

No doubt life in its all forms enjoys a very high status in Islam. Indeed, human life is one of the most sacred creations of God. Therefore, it must be appreciated, respected and protected. This paper presents the topic at hand in two parts. The first part examines the value of life in Islam. It will assist us in understanding why life must be appreciated and respected. The second part examines the way the protection of life is regulated in Islamic law and bioethics. Human life must be regulated according to divine instructions; that is, towards its best and most fully human outcome. The maintenance of physical health and the treatment of the sick are important aspects of Islamic teachings in this regard. In respect to the beginning of human life, first we will see that reproduction must occur in the context of a stable and legitimate family. Second, we will see how abortion is viewed in Islamic law and bioethics. In respect to the end of life, issues such as euthanasia and suicide will be investigated. It will be argued that such acts demonstrate a lack of respect for human life and are morally wrong.

Part I: Respect for Life

Life is a divine quality: Among the attributes and names of God which are mentioned in Islamic scriptures, "the Living" (*al-Hayy*) is one of the most obvious and outstanding. The Qur'an says:

And put your trust in the Living one Who dies not,
and glorify His praise… (25:58)

He is the Living, there is no god but He, therefore
call on Him, being sincere to Him in obedience.
All praise is due to God, the Lord of the worlds.
(40:65)

Sanctity of Life

Life is sacred and is one of the greatest gifts and blessings of
God. Every moment of life has great value and is irreversible.
Therefore, life must be appreciated and protected, even if it is of a
poor quality. All forms of life are precious and are considered to
be signs of God. However, among all the forms of life which
exist in the material world, human life is the most significant and
the most precious. Referring to the different stages in the creation
of mankind, the Qur'an says:

And certainly We created man of an extract of
clay. Then We made him a zygote in a firm
resting-place. Then We made the zygote a clot,
then We made the clot a lump of flesh, then We
made (in) the lump of flesh bones, then We caused
it to grow into another creation, so blessed be God,
the Best of creators. (23:14)

The above verse refers to the different phases of the creation of
man. The first part of the verse, which relates to the creation of
man from soil, refers to the creation of the first man, Adam. The
next part of the verse refers to the creation of Adam's offspring,
generation by generation. Human life has such importance that
God mentions its development step by step. Finally, after
reference to the creation of spirit - which is considered as
"khalqan ākhar" - God says: "Blessed be the Best of creators!"
(23:14) If the creator of man is the best of creators, then man
himself must be the best of creatures - at least potentially.

Therefore, life must be appreciated and respected. Killing an innocent person is not only considered a criminal act (i.e., murder), but also represents an underestimation of and insult to human life as a whole. This fact is interestingly expressed in the following verse:

> For this reason We prescribed to the Children of Israel that whoever slays a soul, unless it be for manslaughter or for mischief in the land, it is as though he slew all men; and whoever keeps it alive, it is as though he kept alive all men; and certainly Our messengers came to them with clear proofs, but even after that many of them certainly act extravagantly in the land. (5:32)

One may conclude from the above verse that:

a. Causing the death of one person unjustifiably is like causing the death of all humanity. In other words, lack of respect for an individual life demonstrates a lack of respect for life as such and, therefore, for all individual lives.[1] This is in addition to the fact that whoever commits a murder is likely to murder more people and endanger humanity.[2]

b. Giving life to someone, or more precisely, saving one person's life out of one's respect for life, is like saving all people (from imminent danger).

c. Causing the death of a murderer or someone who does mischief on earth is permitted since it demonstrates respect for lost life and prevents further danger to society and damage to life as a whole. This is why the Qur'an considers the legislation of retaliation to be something that is needed, though pardon is preferable when there is no fear of threat to the security of the public.[3]

In Islamic law and morality, murder in general, and the murder of believers in particular, is treated very severely; the Qur'an enjoins the everlasting punishment of hell for those who deliberately commit such an act. We also read in Islamic hadiths that the destruction of the whole (physical) world is less vicious in the eyes of God than the murder of an innocent person.

Animal life: We find in Islamic hadiths that even hurting or killing animals unjustifiably is treated very severely. For example, Imam Sadiq, the sixth Imam of the Shi'a, mentioned the Divine punishment of a woman who had fastened a cat with a rope so that the cat could not move and died from thirst.[4] A typical view among the Shi'a jurists can be found in the following passage by 'Allamah Mohammad Taqi Ja'fari:

> Consideration of whole sources of Islamic jurisprudence (*fiqh*) leads to the conclusion that animals must not be killed unless there is a legal permission (by God) like benefiting from them or being safe from their harm. There are adequate reasons for prohibiting hunting animals for fun and one can argue from these reasons for the prohibition of killing animals without having a permitting cause.[5]

The above idea is part of a broader Islamic perspective on the life of animals. According to Islamic law, there are many rights which are reserved for animals that must be observed. The proper consideration of those rights shows that not only must their life be protected, but their quality of life must be safeguarded as well. For example, animals must not be burdened by being forced to carry heavy goods or to move faster than they can tolerate. Nor can animals be treated unjustly by cursing or swearing at them. It is reported that Imam Ali said: "Whoever curses an animal, he himself will be cursed by God."[6]

Who is the giver of life and death? This is one of the basic questions in bioethics which can thoroughly influence one's approach towards life and its regulation. If one believes that life is created by chance, or that it can be created by man himself, then it will lose its sanctity and the end-result would be that it could also be destroyed by either man or chance. But if life is a gift of God, then who are we to take it away?

God is the only source of life. In other words, all forms of life are originated by Him. This is an idea in which special emphasis has been put in the Qur'an. For example, we read:

> Verily, it is God Who causes the seed-grain and the fruit stone (like date-stone) to split and sprout. He brings forth the living from the dead, and it is He Who brings forth the dead from the living. Such is God, then how are you deluded away from the truth? (6:95)

> And a sign for them is the dead land. We give it life, and we bring forth from it grains, so that they eat thereof. (36:33)

Thus, life is a gift of God for which we are held responsible. Not only is it God Who gives life, but it is only God Who can bring life to an end. For example, we read in the Qur'an:

> There is no god but He. It is He who gives life and causes death - your Lord and the Lord of your forefathers. (44:8)

> ...You bring the living out of the dead, and you bring the dead out of the living. And You give sustenance to whom You will, without limit. (3:27)

> It is He Who gives life and causes death. And when He decides upon a thing He says to it only: "Be!" – and it is. (40:68)

19

> Say (to them): "God gives you life, then causes
> you to die, then He will assemble you on the Day
> of Resurrection about which there is no doubt. But
> most of mankind know not." (45:26)[7]

The Qur'an blames those who attribute the cause of death to
going on a journey, fighting, illness or to people themselves.

> O you who believe! Be not like those who
> disbelieve and say about their brethren when they
> travel on the earth or go out to fight: "If they had
> stayed with us, they would not have died or been
> killed," so that God may make it a cause of regret
> in their hearts. It is God that gives life and causes
> death. And God is All-Seer of what you do.
> (3:156)

According to the Qur'an, after refuting Nimrod's claim of deity,
the Prophet Abraham said (to him): "My Lord is He Who gives
life and causes death." (2:258) Nimrod said: "I give life and
cause death." (Ibid) Then Nimrod asked a prisoner who was
supposed to be executed to be released and another prisoner who
was not supposed to be killed to be executed. When Abraham
saw the depth of Nimrod's ignorance and deception about the
real meaning of *giving life* and *causing death,* and the tacit
approval of the people who were present, he said to Nimrod:

> "Verily, God causes the sun to rise from the east;
> then cause it you rise from the west." So the
> disbeliever was utterly defeated. And God does not
> guide the unjust people. (Ibid)

Now, let us reflect on the real meaning of giving life and causing
death. Does it mean that nothing other than God can bear on - or
get involved in - the process of giving life or causing death?
Obviously not. For example, reproduction is certainly a form of
involvement in the process of life. This is also true with regards
to feeding and caring for a child as well. Children feel indebted

towards their parents for their existence. On the other hand, a murderer is held responsible for – in a sense – causing death to his victim.[8] While it is true that Nimrod or even his agents could have had a significant role in the death of their victim, it is still true that *"it is God that gives life and causes death."* (3:156) Likewise, we see this verity again in Abraham's argument against Nimrod that *"My Lord is He Who gives life and causes death."* (2:258)

The great Shi'a exegete of the Qur'an, Sayyid Muhammad Husayn Tabataba'i, writes:

> When Ibrahim [i.e., Abraham] mentioned life and death, he meant life and death as we find them in living things. His argument was that these living things could only be created by One who was the source of life. Lifeless nature cannot bestow life on others when it has no life itself...

> If Namrud [Nimrod] had interpreted Ibrahim's argument honestly, he could not have refuted it at all. But he resorted to deception, interpreting life and death with an allegorical meaning. "To give life" really means, for example, to create a living foetus; but it may be used equally correctly (but in a metaphorical way) if you rescue someone from an extremely dangerous situation. Likewise, "to cause to die" really means the act of God by which a soul departs from a body; but metaphorically it may be used for murder, etc. (14, p. 184)

Thus, it is possible to suppose that man, as well as the natural environment, can have a role in the process of giving life and causing death. The reason is this - *in this world, God usually acts through natural rules and the cause and effect system.*[9] It is also possible to suppose that natural factors and circumstances may have a role in something being created or brought into existence.[10] However, it is only God Who truly and genuinely brings something into existence or gives life.[11] We humans have no control or even complete knowledge of our existence or life. So how is it possible to suppose that we can grant existence or life to something else?

Dignity of Man

In Islam, human beings have an important status. In the Qur'an, man is respected and honoured:

> And surely We have honoured the children of Adam, and We have carried them in the land and the sea, and we have given them to excel by an appropriate excellence over most of those whom we have created. (17:70)

Human beings can act as God's vicegerents on earth. The Qur'an says:

> And when your Lord said to the angels: I am going to place on the earth a vicegerent. (2:30)

> And He it is who has made you vicegerents (inheritors) in the land and raised some of you above others by (various) grades, that He might try you by what He has given you… (6:165)

They are endowed with reason and free will and therefore are responsible for what they do. Therefore, it is only humans who bear the divine trust and can fulfill the goal of creation:

> We offered the trust to the heavens and the earth and the mountains, but they refused to carry it and were afraid of it; and man carried it. Surely he is very unjust, very ignorant. (33:72)

This verse suggests that the main problems that man is faced with when exercising his freewill is injustice and ignorance.[12] Of course, God has provided human beings with the basic knowledge required to distinguish between what is (morally) good or bad:

> And inspired it what is wrong for it and (what is) right for it. (91:8)

> We showed him the Way: whether he be grateful or ungrateful (rests on his will). (76:3)

Man & the world: Man can benefit from nature, and indeed, every blessing of God, including their own bodies and souls, in a responsible way. Thus we read in the Qur'an:

> And He has subjected to you, as from Him, all that is in the heavens and on earth: Behold, in that are Signs indeed for those who reflect. (45:13)

> It is He Who hath created for you all things that are on earth... (2:29)

> Then on that day you shall most certainly be questioned about the blessings. (102:8)

Therefore, everything in the world which is at our disposal is both a gift and a trust. If these things were merely a trust, then we would not have permission to use them. Yet since they are gifts of God, we are able to make use of them. However, we cannot be wasteful or extravagant, as is the case with any trust.

> And He it is Who produces gardens (of vine), trellised and untrellised, and palms and seed-produce of which the fruits are of various sorts, and olives and pomegranates, like and unlike; eat of its fruit when it bears fruit, and pay the due of it on the day of its reaping, and do not act extravagantly; surely He does not love the extravagant. (6:141)

> O Children of Adam! Wear your beautiful apparel
> at every time and place of prayer: eat and drink,
> but waste not by excess, for God does not love the
> wasteful. (7:31)

In addition to this, the Qur'an tells us that we are supposed to make efforts to improve environmental conditions as much as possible:

> He brought you forth from the earth and has asked
> you to improve it, therefore ask forgiveness of
> Him, then turn to Him; surely my Lord is Nigh,
> Answering. (11:61)

Therefore, we must be very careful about the way we treat nature, other human beings and ourselves.

Dignity of body and soul: We should always remember that, in Islam, there is a close link between the body and the soul, or between the material and the spiritual. In the same way that we need to look after our physical health, we need to look after our spiritual health and vice versa. The dignity of man extends to his body and thus there is no way to harm the human body or treat it with disrespect.

This dignity also extends to the period after death.[13] There are many rulings pertaining to the human corpse, which all indicate the continuity of the respect given to the human body even after the separation of spirit. For example, the human corpse must be properly washed, dressed, prayed for and buried. The body must be buried in a respected place and the direction of Mecca must be observed. It is not permissible to exhume graves or unveil a buried body.[14] Autopsy is allowed, but only if absolutely necessary (for example, when there is suspicion of murder).[15]

According to many hadiths, the performance of any act that causes death to a living person, like cutting off someone's head, is forbidden, even if it is performed on a dead person.[16] Indeed, it is considered to be the most horrible act of all since the dead have no power to defend themselves.[17]

Part II: Protection for Life

Islamic guidance on practical issues related to life in general, and human life in particular, can be sought in the field of Islamic bioethics. As we will see later, because of the interconnectedness of Islamic law and ethics, Islamic bioethics has to consider the requirements of Islamic law (*shari'ah*) in addition to various moral considerations. As a result, everything has to be double-checked - first against legal standards and then against moral standards. It seems that many of those who have written on Islamic bioethics have not made a distinction between the two. Although it is certainly true that there is absolute harmony and compatibility between Islamic law and morality, their aims and objectives are different and, therefore, they may differ in their prescriptions. For example, one difference is that while Islamic law tries to meet minimum requirements for the perfection or happiness in both worlds - which are manageable for the average or even lower than average person - Islamic ethics tries to show people who have greater ambitions how to become more perfect and closer to God.

Therefore, whatever is deemed necessary or obligatory in Islamic law is certainly the same in Islamic ethics. However, there may be cases which are not explicitly prohibited in Islamic law, which, at the same time, may be condemned within the Islamic ethical system. Or there may be cases which are not compulsory in Islamic law, but are necessary from an ethical point of view. For instance, while idle chatter is not prohibited in Islamic law, it is considered a waste of precious time as well as harmful to spiritual development, and thus is ethically condemned. Another example is the night prayers (which should be performed after midnight and before dawn). Night prayers are highly recommended, but are not mandatory within Islamic law.

However, Muslim ethicists and spiritual masters normally uphold the idea that they are necessary for those who aspire to greater spiritual heights and who are striving for spiritual perfection. Elsewhere, I have written:

> So *fiqh* mainly comprises basic and necessary laws whose obedience is required from all Muslims, and is considered the first step towards development. To commit oneself to the laws of *fiqh* is not a difficult undertaking, as Islam itself is not a difficult religion. However, there always are individuals who observe the mandatory laws of *fiqh,* yet upon getting a glimpse of the Light, want nothing more than to fly to the Flame. For these enraptured souls, Islam has provided *akhlaq.* They then make mandatory upon themselves deeds which are highly recommended, or *mustahab.* In addition to performing these recommended tasks, they obey other laws of *akhlaq,* and make unlawful upon themselves that which is not forbidden in *fiqh,* yet somehow might be an obstacle on the way to the Light, to perfection.[18]

Therefore, if issues such as abortion are prohibited in Islamic law, then it follows that it is certainly prohibited in the Islamic ethical system as well. However, it is quite possible to think that while something like cloning may be permissible from a legal point of view, it may still be morally challenged.

Thus, in order to discover the basis of Islamic bioethics, we need to reflect on the rulings of Islamic law, as well as the prescriptions of Islamic ethics, in order to find out the benefits which they try to secure and the harms which they try to prevent. Moral considerations must not be overshadowed by incorporating a solely legal approach, just as legal requirements cannot be compromised either.

Sources of Islamic Bioethics

Like any other enquiry about Islam, Islamic bioethics is based on the Qur'an, the Sunnah and reason. Instead of employing reason, Sunni Muslims may refer to things like *ijmā'* (consensus), *qiyās* (analogy) and *istihsān* (discretion). For the Shi'a, *ijmā'*, *qiyās* and *istihsān* as such are not accepted, since they by themselves cannot prove anything. On the whole, the bioethical rulings of the Shi'a and the Sunni schools of thought do not fundamentally differ, especially in respect to those problems for which direct guidance has been received from the Qur'an and Sunnah. When problems become more speculative, however, the positions are more likely to differ.

Where does authority lie in Islamic bioethics?

In Shi'a Islam, the determination of valid religious practice is reserved for the Grand Ayatollahs (*marāji'* of *taqlid*), who are the most qualified jurisprudents of each generation. They provide rulings on whether a given action is forbidden, discouraged, neutral, recommended or obligatory. It should be noted that every Ayatollah is required to refer directly to the main sources, i.e., the Qur'an, the Sunnah and reason, in order to discover the correct Islamic teachings in each case. Although he carefully and respectfully studies the works of his predecessors, an Ayatollah must develop his own original understanding and must not follow any other Ayatollah, however great the other *marāji'* may have been. As I mentioned above, even consensus among people or among other scholars is, by itself, not a proof. This situation has provided a kind of dynamism and vitality to Shi'a thought. Elsewhere I have written:

> Thus, for the Shi'a, consensus in itself is not a proof. It only works when it leads to the discovery of Sunnah. Accordingly, if Muslims today agree on a given subject, while a scholar has doubt about the Islamic judgement on that subject, he methodologically cannot say that because

everybody says so, I also say the same. There have been many cases in history where all human beings believed in the same way and later they found out that they were wrong, e.g., the earth being flat. It is only the Qur'an and the Sunnah that are unquestionably true and immune from any error or mistake. This approach grants a type of dynamism to Shi'i thought, so that every generation of scholars, and even any single scholar, is able, and indeed is required, to refer directly to the Qur'an and Sunnah and conduct his own original *ijtihād,* that is his investigation and independent judgement. *Ijtihād* has never been banned or closed in the Shi'a world. The Shi'a believe that the view of no jurist, however high his position, is immune from scientific questioning or challenge. Of course, as in any other discipline, every religious scholar needs to consult and examine carefully the works of his predecessors.[19]

What is the basis of Islamic bioethics?

If secular Western bioethics is mostly based upon individual rights, what is the basis of Islamic bioethics? It has been suggested that "Islamic bioethics is based on duties and obligations (e.g., to preserve life, seek treatment), although rights (of God, the community and the individual) do feature in bioethics, as does a call to virtue (*Ihsān*)."[20] I think it is true that Islamic bioethics is expressed primarily as duties and obligations. However, it should be noted that, in Islamic bioethics, we have to meet legal requirements, and therefore, we try to infer our duties and obligations from the original sources. In other words, emphasis is normally put upon duties and obligations. However, there seems to be no doubt that Islamic legislation is altogether intended to secure our interests. God, the Almighty, does not gain anything if we obey Him. Neither does He lose anything if we disobey Him. It is only out of His wisdom and mercy that He has provided us with a legal system, which includes commands and prohibitions, so that we know what benefits us or harms us in this world and the Hereafter. Thus, every obligation from God is indeed a guidance towards some interest/s that one has the right to have.

Issues in Bioethics

I. Treatment of the Sick

Islam emphasises the importance of maintaining one's health and preventing illness, but when prevention fails, all efforts must be made to restore health. One way to save lives is to treat people when they become sick. It is a mutual responsibility of the sick and the physicians (or society in general). In other words, seeking treatment is a duty for the sick person and everybody within the society is obliged to help the sick in their treatment as well. On the necessity of treatment, the Prophet said:

> O Servants of Allah, seek treatment, for Allah has not sent down any illness without sending down its treatment.[21]

This is a sample of a set of narrations that makes treatment mandatory when a specific treatment is available, and also if holding off this treatment would be harmful. On the other hand, healing people is considered to be a sacred job. The physician must do his best to heal the sick, but at the same time he must know that the real healer is God. In the Qur'an, Prophet Abraham is quoted as saying: *"And when I am sick, He restores me to health."* (26: 80) Indeed, one of the names of God is "the Healer" (*al-Shafi*).

The physician must also treat the patient with respect and compassion. The Oath of the Muslim Doctor includes an undertaking "to protect human life in all stages and under all circumstances, doing [one's] utmost to rescue it from death, malady, pain and anxiety. To be, all the way, an instrument of God's mercy, extending...medical care to near and far, virtuous and sinner and friend and enemy." [22]

II. Reproduction

Due to the high value of human life, Islam attaches special attention to life before it begins and even after it ends with death. The only proper and legitimate way for having a child is through marriage. In other words, a male and female may have a child only when they appreciate the value of human life and are committed to taking the full responsibility of bringing up a child in the sacred institution of the family. Marriage is not just a financial or physical arrangement for having sexual relations or living together under one roof. Nor is it just a legal contract between a man and woman. Marriage is a sacred covenant between two parties with God as its witness. Marriage is a gift of God for human beings to complement and console themselves with each other. The Qur'an says:

> Among His signs is [the fact] that He has created spouses for you from among yourselves so that you may console yourselves with them. He has planted affection and mercy between you; in that are signs for people who contemplate. (30:21)

> God has granted you spouses from among yourselves, and granted you children and grandchildren by means of your spouses. He has provided you with wholesome things. So will they still believe in vain things and be ungrateful to God's favour? (16:72)

Violation of this sacred covenant by adultery or by homosexual relations is unlawful and is unanimously rejected by all Muslim scholars. It is also immoral to use modern biotechnology to bypass marriage and reproduce artificially out of the context of the family. Of course, a married couple may use legitimate biomedical techniques for parenting. The Qur'an says:

30

He is the One Who created humanity from water.
Then he established blood ties as well as in-laws.
(25:54)

III. Family Planning

Islam considers having children as a great gift of God and highly
recommends people to get married and establish family ties and
have children. However, Islam does not compel people to get
married or have children after marriage unless there is an
overriding (secondary) reason which makes marriage and the
formation of a family or having children necessary. For example, if
the only way to protect one's piety and chastity is to get married or
if the protection of the people of faith from the attacks of enemies
depends on the increase in the number of the members of the
society, it becomes compulsory to get married and have children.[23]

Thus, Islam allows family planning to prevent pregnancy, but does
not allow the termination of pregnancy.[24] Now, naturally the
question arises as to when pregnancy starts and whether the
beginning of pregnancy coincides with the beginning of human life
or not.

IV. Abortion

Islam prohibits abortion unless there is an exceptional situation
for which the *shari'ah* permits it as a lesser evil.[25] A typical
Islamic point of view can be found in the following statement by
the Islamic Organization for Medical Sciences:

> **One:** The inception of life occurs with the union of
> a sperm and an ovum, forming a zygote which
> carries the full genetic code of the human race in
> general and of the particular individual, who is
> different from all others throughout the ages. The
> zygote begins a process of cleavage that yields a
> growing and developing embryo, which progresses
> through the stages of gestation towards birth.

31

Two: From the moment a zygote settles inside a woman's body, it deserves a unanimously recognized degree of respect, and a number of legal stipulations, known to all scholars, apply to it.

Three: When it arrives at the spirit-breathing stage...the foetus acquires greater sanctity, as all scholars agree, and additional legal stipulations apply to it.[26]

Abortion, especially after the spirit is blown into the foetus, is considered to be an act of infanticide and the Qur'anic condemnation of killing one's children would then apply. Regarding infanticide, the Qur'an states:

Kill not your children for fear of want. We shall provide sustenance for them as well as for you. Verily the killing of them is a great sin. (17:31)

Kill not your children on a plea of want. We will provide sustenance for you and for them. Come not near shameful deeds whether open or secret. Take not life which God has been made sacred except by way of justice and law. Thus He commands you that you may learn wisdom. (6:151)

The pledge of the believing women that they shall not kill their children. (60:12)

And when the female infant who was buried alive is asked for what crime she was killed? (81:8-9)

Islam severely condemned the practice of the pagans who killed their children due to poverty or because of the shame of the birth of a girl. Unfortunately, today we see millions of abortions take place every year. Most of these abortions take place because the so-called "liberated" people of our age would like to enjoy a life of sexual freedom. These are the people "who have taken their religion (way of life) to be mere amusement and play and were deceived by the worldly life." (7:51)

When does the prohibition of abortion apply?

The general Islamic view is that, although there is some form of life which exists after conception, human life fully begins only after the ensoulment of the foetus. Most Muslim scholars, including the Shi'a, believe that ensoulment occurs at about 120 days after conception.[27] There is a minority that hold that it occurs at about 40 days after conception. Of course, as soon as the zygote settles inside a woman's body, it deserves a unanimously recognized degree of respect and cannot be aborted. The Qur'an uses the word "haml" to describe pregnancy.[28] In Arabic, the term "haml" means to carry and this starts when the zygote is implanted in the uterus. The late Ayatollah Khu'i said: "The criterion in applying the [word] 'pregnant' for a woman is correct only after the settling down (istiqrār) of the zygote in her womb because just the entering of the sperm in her womb does not make her pregnant."[29]

Thus, from the very beginning of the pregnancy, its termination is prohibited and the zygote must be protected. The respect shown to the zygote at this early stage does not necessarily mean that it is a real or actual human being.[30] After pregnancy starts, the zygote is in a state of active potentiality to become a human being with the full genetic code of the human race in general and of the particular individual. As we saw above in the verse 23:13, the implantation of the ovum in the uterus constitutes the first stage of the creation of man. According to a hadith, Ishaq b. 'Ammar asked Imam al-Kazim (a) whether or not it was permissible for a woman who feared she was pregnant to drink some liquid to abort what was in her uterus. Imam replied: "No." Ishaq said: "That is the zygote (nutfah)." Imam replied: "Verily the first thing to be created is the zygote."[31] However, it is only later, when the spirit is created, that it becomes a real human being. For this reason, Shi'a jurists, like the late Ayatollah Khomeini, Ayatollah Khamenei, Ayatollah

Lankarani and Ayatollah Sistani, declare that it is allowed to abort a foetus to save the life of the mother before the ensoulment of the child. However, after ensoulment has taken place, it is prohibited to sacrifice the foetus for the sake of the mother.[32]

In his famous medical work entitled *The Canon of Medicine,* Ibn Sina studies the techniques of bringing the embryo out of the womb.[33] Although his discussion is medical in nature rather than jurisprudential, he makes it very clear that such operations can only take place in clearly defined situations when there is no other option. In order to prevent any misuse by those who may want to perform abortions, he asserts that such operations can be performed only in the following circumstances:

1- When the mother is too young and cannot bear pregnancy and would certainly die during delivery. In this case, in order to save her life, the embryo must be removed before its growth has been completed.

2- When the mother's womb is damaged and extra flesh has blocked the path for delivery. Such a child would not survive the delivery and would die in its mother's womb.

3- The child has already died in the womb. In this case, efforts must be made to remove the dead body of the unborn child.

He adds that, if the mother has labour pains for four days and the child has not been born, it must be assumed that the child has died and one must do their best to save the mother rather than attempt to rescue the child. The techniques that he mentions for removing the child basically involve certain movements carried out by the mother as well as dietary and medicinal methods.[34]

V. Death

Islam places great emphasis on the sanctity of life while highlighting the reality of death at the same time. Indeed, to have a better appreciation of life, one needs to remember death and its inevitability. It is only then that one realizes that one must make optimal benefit of one's life. Thus, unlike what many people think today, Islam considers the remembrance of death as a source of vitality and spiritual power. About one third of the Qur'an talks about Resurrection, death and the life after death. For example, we read:

> Every soul shall have a taste of death. (2:35)

> No soul can die except by God's permission. (3:185)

"Everyone is created for a life span and dying is a part of the contract (with God) and the final decision (of term) is up to God. The quality of life is equally or more important than the duration of living."[35] In his supplication for acquiring a noble character (*Makārim al-Akhlāq*), Imam Sajjad, the fourth Imam of the Shi'a, asks God:

> Let me live as long as my life is used is serving Thee. When my life becomes a pasture for Satan, be pleased to call me back to Thee before Thy wrath advances towards me or Thy anger be fixed upon me.

Death consists in the separation of the soul from the body. However, the exact time of this separation cannot be known with certainty like the time of ensoulment. Therefore, death is diagnosed by its physical signs. However, when there is doubt, maximum caution must be taken into account. It should be noted that there is a difference between reaching an irreversible state in which death becomes decisive and actually dying. Second, if a person still shows some vital signs, such as a heartbeat, and even if (and this is really an if) we can scientifically know that his soul has departed from his body, nothing must be done in order to hasten death or commit a disrespectful act to human life.

It seems to me that one should be able to distinguish between saving a life (which is compulsory in Islam) through medical treatment, financial support or otherwise and artificially prolonging life.[36] For example, if someone is definitely dying because of an advanced cancer and there is no cure, the most that could be done in this situation is to use some medicine to keep him alive for a few days. The cost of this medicine, however, is so high that the whole family would be put into great difficulty by obtaining it. Is it necessary for the patient, his relatives or others to take this measure? Or if this could be performed by a very painful operation, is it necessary for the patient to undergo such an operation when there is no possibility of cure? It seems reasonable to suggest that "the physician and the family should realize their limitations and not attempt heroic measures for a terminally ill patient or to prolong artificially the life (or misery). The heroic measures taken at the beginning of life (i.e., saving a premature baby) may be more justified than at the end of a life span, though each case has to be individualized."[37]

VI. Suicide

If we have not created our life and it is a gift from God for which we are held responsible, it is obvious that we have no absolute power over our lives. Life is a trust from God and we must take care of it to the best of our ability. This is the case with all blessings of God, whether they are physical or spiritual. We can benefit from what we have been given, but we cannot destroy or waste it. No one should say to themselves that they would like to harm their property, health or reputation. Our situation in this world is like a guest who is invited to a guesthouse. Whatever is in the guesthouse is put there by the host for the benefit of the guest. However, the guest cannot burn himself inside the house or destroy the guesthouse or the things which have been put there. This comparison becomes more interesting if we augment this notion with the idea that our body is like a guestroom for our spirit and we must observe the regulations for using this room which have been set out by God. We must try to please God by preserving life and health, promoting a high quality of life and alleviating suffering.

VII. Euthanasia

Islam is against euthanasia (mercy killing). Muslim jurists regard euthanasia as an act of murder. Murder can be performed with a gun or a syringe, by a serial killer or a physician, or even by the victim himself. For example, Ayatollah Khomeini declared that any measure which is utilised for hastening the death of someone is considered to be an act of murder.[38] Ayatollah Makarim Shirazi proclaims that:

> Killing a human being, even out of mercy (euthanasia), or with the consent of the patient, is not allowed.[39]

He argues that the main argument for such prohibition is that the verses and hadiths which indicate the prohibition of murder (*qatl*) apply to such cases. The philosophy beyond this prohibition may be the fact that permitting such acts leads to many misuses and acts of euthanasia or suicide may take place for any weak or trivial excuse. Moreover, medical judgements are usually not definitive and there have been cases in which people who had no hope for recovery were mysteriously saved from death.

VIII. Organ Transplantation

Organ transplantation is practised in almost all Muslim countries. Three situations can be conceived of here:

a) The donor is alive and is willing to donate his organs. This is normally allowed, provided that such donation does not pose any danger to his own life. For example, a healthy person can donate one kidney to another person and still live reasonably well. Indeed, this act may become obligatory when it turns out to be the only way to save a life and organ donation will not put him in an unbearable situation or create any kind of harm for him. One cannot therefore donate any organ on which one's life depends, like the heart or brain.[40]

b) As mentioned above, Islam has a high regard for the dead and this determines many religious and moral decisions regarding cadavers. However, many Muslim scholars have permitted the donation of cadavers, if the person made this decision before his death or his guardian (*wasiyy*) approves of the donation.[41]

c) Donation after brain death: This very much depends on whether or not we accept legal brain death as death or not. Therefore, it will be reduced either to **a** or **b**. Normally, Shi'a scholars, like Ayatollah Khamenei, Ayatollah Bahjat, and Ayatollah Tabrizi, out of maximum care for human life, do not allow any kind of transplant that might lead to the termination of life even in this state and even if the donor has put in his will that his organs can be given to those in need after his death.[42]

Bibliography

Dār, Abdallah S. & Khitamy A. (2001), "Bioethics for Clinicians: 21. Islamic bioethics" in *CMAJ*, January 9.

Gharawi, Mirza 'Ali (1988), *Al-Tanqih fi Sharh-i al-'Urwat al-Wuthqā*, vol. 7 (Najaf: al-Adab Press).

Hurr al-'Amili, Muhammad (1392 A.H), *Wasā'il al-Shi'ah*, section on *Diyat al-a'ḍā*, Chapter 25 (Qum: Ismā'iliyan).

Ibn Sina (1987), *Al-Qānun fi al-Tibb*, Section Three. Translated into Farsi by A. Sharaf Kandi (Tehran: Sorush).

Ja'fari, Mohammad Taqi (2002), *Rasā'il Fiqhi* (Tehran: Tahdhib & Mu'assise-ye 'Allamah Ja'fari).

Karami, Khuda Bandeh (2002), *Euthanasia: Marg-e Asān va Rāhat* (Tehran: Ma'ārif).

Khamenei, Sayyid Ali, *Practical Laws of Islam (Ajwibat al-Istifta'āt)* (Tehran: Islamic Culture and Relations Organization).

Majlesi, Muhammad Baqir (1983), *Bihār al-Anwār* (Beirut: Al-Wafā).

Rizvi, Sayyid Mohammad (1990), *Marriage and Morals in Islam* (Scarborough: Islamic Education & Information Centre).

Rouhani, Mohammad & Nughani, Fatimah (1987), *Ahkām-e Pezeshki* (Tehran: Teymurzadeh).

Shomali, Mohamamd Ali (2004), "Value of Life in Islam" in *Catholics and Shi'a in Dialogue: Studies in Theology & Spirituality* (London: Melisende, 2004).

Shomali, Mohammad Ali (2006), *Self-Knowledge*, 2nd edition (Qum: Jami'at al-Zahra).

Shomali, Mohammad Ali (2007), *Discovering Shi'a Islam*, 6th Edition (London: Islamic Centre of England).

Tabataba'i, Sayyid Muhammad Husayn (1982), *Al-Mizān fi Tafsir al-Qur'an*, vol. 4, translated by Sayyid Akhtar Rizvi (Tehran: WOFIS).

Tabataba'i, Sayyid Muhammad Husayn (1982), *Al-Mizān fi Tafsir al-Qur'an*, vol. 8, translated by Sayyid Akhtar Rizvi (Tehran: WOFIS).

Tabataba'i, Sayyid Muhammad Husayn (2001), *Al-Mizān fi Tafsir al-Qur'an*, vol. 10, translated by Sayyid Akhtar Rizvi (Tehran: WOFIS).

Web sources:

The Full Minutes of the Seminar on "Human Life: Its Inception and End as Viewed by Islam," held on January 15, 1985 CE in Kuwait (http://www.islamset.com/bioethics/incept.html).

"Declaration on Islamic Human Rights," 1990 CE, OIC (Organization of Islamic Conference).

Athar, Shahid, "Islamic Perspectives in Medical Ethics" at http://islam-usa.com/im18.html.

---

[1] Commenting on the above verse, 'Allamah Tabataba'i writes:

> The Divine words: *"Whoever slays a soul...it is as though he slew all men,"* is an allusion to the fact that all men have one single reality, that is, humanity in which all are united, and one and all are equal in it; whoever attacks the humanity found in one of them, he attacks the humanity found in all of them." (vol. 10, p. 146)

> It is narrated in both *Al-Kāfi* and *Ma'āni al-Akhbār* that the fifth Imam of the Shi'a, Imam al-Bāqir (a), was asked: "How can it be as though he slew all men, while he had slain a single soul?" The Imam replied: "He will be put in a place in *Jahannam* (*Gehenna*) where the punishment of the people of the Fire reaches its utmost limit; if he had killed all men, he would have entered the same place." The narrator again asked: "Then if he killed another (man)?" Imam replied: "The punishment will be increased for him." According to the above-quoted verse, the previously mentioned hadith, as well as other hadiths, 'Allamah Tabataba'i concludes that "equality is in the nature of punishment and difference will be in intensity of punishment and the effect it will have on the killer." (Ibid., p. 152)

[2] According to a hadith from the Prophet Muhammad (s), the heart of man admits aspiration and fear unless he sheds blood unjustifiably. When he sheds blood unjustly, his heart turns upside down and becomes very dark so that he does not recognize [what is] good nor does he condemn evil. (Tabataba'i, cited in *Kanz al-'Ummāl*, no. 39951)

[3] For example, see the Qur'an (2:178-79).

[4] Majlesi, Muhammad Baqir (1983), *Bihār al-Anwār* (Beirut: Al-Wafā), vol. 76, p. 136.

[5] Ja'fari, Muhammad Taqi (2002), *Rasā'il Fiqhi* (Tehran: Tahdhib & Mu'assise-ye 'Allamah Ja'fari), p. 250. Elsewhere he writes: "Hunting animals for amusement and without need is prohibited. Therefore, if someone makes a trip for such a [kind of] hunting, his trip is a sinful trip." (Ibid., p. 118)

[6] Ibid., cited from Hurr al-'Amili, Muhammad (1392 A.H), *Wasā'il al-Shi'ah*, section on *Diyat al-a'ḍā*, Chapter 25 (Qum: Ismā'iliyan), vol. 8, p. 356.

[7] There are many more verses which refer to the fact that life and death are exclusively created by God, such as: 3:156, 9:117, 10:31, 22:6, 30:4, 50:43, 53:44, 57:2, 67:2.

[8] Furthermore, whoever can save an innocent life but remains indifferent and allows the person to die is morally responsible.

[9] Of course, there have been miracles and extraordinary acts performed by the Prophets or other holy people. These phenomena may seem to contradict the general rule which was mentioned above: "In this world, God usually acts through natural rules and the cause and effect system." However, it must be noted first that miraculous and extraordinary acts do not represent the usual procedure, and that even in the case of such acts, there is no exception to the cause and effect system. The only difference is that, instead of natural causes, supernatural causes are used. Just as there are natural causes, say, for the treatment of an ill person, there may be supernatural causes, such as prayer and giving charity.

[10] Muslim philosophers divide beings into two main groups: beings of the Universe of Command (*'ālam al-amr*) and beings of the Universe of Creation (*'ālam al-khalq*). For the existence of the first group, there is no need for material conditions. This is related to abstract beings (*al-mujarradāt*) whose creation only depends on God's command, "Be!" For the existence of the latter, material conditions are needed. This is related to material beings (*al-mādiyyāt*), whether they be material only in the beginning or if they remain material forever. Here Divine command for their existence is not issued before completion of the necessary conditions, such as the existence of an apple after the existence of natural conditions like water, heat and light or after the existence of supernatural conditions. In other words, for the creation or existence of the first group, it is only an originating cause (*al-'illah al-fā'iliyyah*) which is needed, but for the creation of the latter group, both originating cause and material cause (*al-'illah al-mādiyyah*) are needed.

[11] It has to be noted that God may revive something by the hand of whom He is pleased with. For example, the Qur'an talks about Abraham who was shown

how God gives life to the dead. (2:260) Another example is Jesus, who was able to *"bring the dead to life with God's permission."* (3:49)

[12] Injustice is a very broad concept and includes any act of disobedience to God or any act of harm to one's self or others: *"Every person who breaks divine laws has oppressed himself."* (95:61) If a person does not pray or fast, then he has been unjust to himself. When a person beats someone or robs him of his money, he is initially doing a disservice to himself, then to the other person. Committing a sin is just like drinking poisoned water. Now if this person drinks poison, he is hurting himself. The same logic can be applied when he harms another being. The consequences of his ill acts would be his destroying the bases of his inherent God-given purity. He initiates hindrances on the way to his perfection.

[13] Hurr al-'Amili, Muhammad (1392 A.H), *Wasā'il al-Shi'ah*, section on *Diyat al-a'da*, Chapter 25 (Qum: Ismā'iliyān).

[14] In his reply to Question 1277 in *Ajwibat al-Istifta'āt*, Ayatollah Khamenei does not allow the graves of Muslims to be dug up in order to exhume their bones for training purposes in schools of medicine unless there is a pressing medical need for the bones and it is impossible to obtain them otherwise. Upon reflection, we may conclude that if there are non-Muslims who are willing to sell or give the bones of their dead free of charge, then Muslims must approach them as non-Muslims would not consider this to be a disrespectful act towards their dead.

[15] Q1274: Is it permissible to carry out a post-mortem examination to determine the cause of death in doubtful cases, e.g., we do not know whether it happened due to poison, suffocation, or something else?
A: If getting to the truth hinges upon it, there is no objection to it. (*Ajwibat al-Istifta'āt*)

[16] For example, Husayn b. Khalid says that Abu 'Abdillah (Imam Sadiq, the sixth Imam) was asked about a man who cut off the head of a corpse. Imam replied: "Verily God has prohibited in respect to someone when he is dead the same thing that He has prohibited when he is alive. So whoever does to a dead person what causes death to a living person must pay *diyah* (blood money) in its entirety. I asked Abu al-Hasan (the seventh Imam, Imam Kazim) about this. Imam replied: "Abu 'Abdillah told the truth. The Prophet had said this." I said: "So whoever cuts off the head of a corpse or chops open his stomach or does anything else that causes death to the living must pay the *diyah* of a complete person?" Imam replied: "He must pay the *diyah* of an embryo in the womb of his mother before the spirit is created into it and that is 100 *dinār* (golden coin). The *diyah* of the embryo belongs to his heirs, but the *diyah* of this dead person belongs to him and not to the heirs." I asked: "What is the difference between them?" Imam replied: "Verily the embryo is something prospective

whose benefit is hoped for (sought), while the dead is something which has expired and whose benefit has gone. Therefore, when his organs are severed (*muthlah*) after his death, the *diyah* belongs to himself and not to others. With this money, hajj (pilgrimage to Mecca) will be performed on his behalf and different types of good deeds like giving alms will be done." [Majlesi, Muhammad Baqir (1983), *Bihār al-Anwār* (Beirut: Al-Wafā), vol. 101, p. 425, Hadith No. 5. See also Ibid., vol. 48, p. 75.]

[17] See e.g. *Wasā'il al-Shi'ah*, section on *Diyat al-a'da*, Chapter 25 (Qum: Ismā'iliyān).

[18] 12, p. 34.

[19] Shomali, M. A. (2007), *Discovering Shi'a Islam*, 6th Edition (Qum: Jami'at al-Zahra) pp. 40-41.

[20] "Bioethics for Clinicians: 21. Islamic bioethics" by Abdallah S. Dār and A. Khitamy in CMAJ, January 9, 2001.

[21] Majlesi, Muhammad Baqir (1983), *Bihār al-Anwār* (Beirut: Al-Wafā), vol. 59, p. 76.

[22] "Bioethics for clinicians: 21. Islamic bioethics" by Abdallah S. Dār and A. Khitamy in CMAJ, January 9, 2001.

[23] In *Marriage and Morals in Islam* (Scarborough: Islamic Education & Information Centre), Chapter Four, S.M. Rizvi writes:

> According to the Shi 'ah fiqh, family planning as a private measure to space or regulate the family size for health or economic reasons is permissible. Neither is there any Qur'anic verse or hadith against birth control, nor is it *wājib* [obligatory] to have children in marriage. So basically, birth control would come under the category of *jā'iz*, lawful acts. Moreover, we have some *ahadith* (especially on the issue of *'azl, coitus interruptus*) which categorically prove that birth control is permissible.

Later, he adds that "the majority of our *mujtahids* believe that *coitus interruptus* is allowed but *makruh* [disliked] without the wife's consent." (*Sharh al-Lum'ah*, vol. 2, p. 28; *Al-'Urwah*, p. 628; *Minhaj*, vol. 2, p. 267)

[24] Family planning in itself is not forbidden, but there are certain methods of family planning which are not allowed. These details are discussed by Muslim jurists.

[25] For example, see Article 1.e of OIC (Organization of Islamic Conference) Declaration on Islamic Human Rights, 1990.

[26] The Full Minutes of the Seminar on "Human Life: Its Inception and End as Viewed by Islam", Held on January 15, 1985 A.D. in Kuwait. (http://www.islamset.com/bioethics/incept.html). It has to be noted that although this organization mainly follows the Sunni interpretation of Islamic law, what has been mentioned above is, in general, acceptable to both Sunni and Shi'a Muslims.

[27] For example, see Majlesi, Muhammad Baqir (1983), *Bihār al-Anwār* (Beirut: Al-Wafā), vol. 101, p. 425. My humble view is that the reason for fixing the period after 120 days as the time of ensoulment is to provide a practical guideline for settling cases in which parents or medical staff need to make a quick medical decision. Otherwise, in reality, it may be possible that, in some cases, ensoulment could take place slightly later.

[28] See the verses 19:22; 31:14; 46:15.

[29] Rizvi, Sayyid Mohammad (1990), *Marriage and Morals in Islam* (Scarborough: Islamic Education & Information Centre) cited from al-Gharawi, Mirza Ali, *Al-Tanqih fi Sharh-i al-'Urwat al-Wuthqā* (notes from the *fiqh* lectures of Ayatollah al-Khu'i), vol. 7, p. 206 (Najaf: al-Adab Press, 1988). S. M. Rizvi adds that, in 1987, he wrote to Ayatollah al-Khu'i asking him whether it is permissible to use a medicine or a device which prevents the fertilized ovum from implanting itself onto the wall of the uterus. The Ayatollah replied that it is forbidden to abort the zygote after its settling down [in the uterus], whereas [to prevent pregnancy] before that [point] is alright.

[30] As we saw earlier in the discussion about animal life, the necessity of respect for life is not limited to human life alone.

[31] Hurr al-'Amili, Muhammad (1392 A.H), *Wasā'il al-Shi'ah*, Section on *Diyat al-a'ḍā*, Chapter 25 (Qum: Ismā'iliyan), vol. 19, p. 15.

[32] Rouhani, Mohammad & Nughani, Fatimah (1987), *Ahkām-e Pezeshki* (Tehran: Teymurzadeh), pp. 107-125.

[33] *The Canon of Medicine (Al-Qānun fi al-tibb)* is a book by the great Persian philosopher, scientist and physician, Ibn Sina. The book was based on both his own personal experience and medieval Islamic medicine in general as well as traditional Persian and Arabian medicine. It is considered to be one of the most famous books in the history of medicine and remained a pre-eminent medical authority for centuries.

[34] Ibn Sina (1987), *Al-Qānun fi al-Tibb*, Section Three. Translated into Farsi by A. Sharaf Kandi (Tehran: Sorush), section 3, p. 327.

[35] Athar, Shahid Athar, "Islamic Perspectives in Medical Ethics" at http://islam-usa.com/im18.htm.

[36] This is the author's humble view which he takes to be in compliance with the views of Muslim jurists. However, the issue needs further investigation.

[37] Athar, Shahid Athar, "Islamic Perspectives in Medical Ethics" at http://islam-usa.com/im18.htm.

[38] Rouhani, Mohammad & Nughani, Fatimah (1987), *Ahkām-e Pezeshki* (Tehran: Teymurzadeh), p. 180.

[39] Ibid.

[40] Q1279: If a person is suffering from a fatal illness and doctors say he will die soon, is it permissible to remove certain organs from his body, such as the heart, kidney, etc., before he is dead so that it can be transplanted into the body of another person?

A: If the removal of the organs from the patient's body leads to his death, it amounts to murder. Otherwise, there is no objection to it provided that it is done with the person's permission.

Q1283: Since having a kidney transplant would improve the patient's condition considerably, there has been an intention to set up a kidney bank. This is bound to encourage people to donate or sell their kidneys willingly. Is it permissible to donate or sell one's body part by choice, whether it is a kidney or any other organ? And what is the ruling in emergency conditions?

A: There is no objection to the living *mukallaf* donating or selling his organs in order that the sick may make use of them provided that he will not be considerably harmed. Indeed, this becomes obligatory when it becomes the only way to save a respected life [as long as] he is not going to put himself in an unbearable situation and it is not harmful for him. [Khamenei, Sayyid Ali, *Practical Laws of Islam (Ajwibat al-Istifta'āt)* (Tehran: Islamic Culture and Relations Organization)]

[41] Q1280: Is it permissible to use the blood vessels of a dead person for transplantation into the body of another person who is ill?

A: There is no objection to it provided that it is done with the permission of the person in their lifetime, or with that of their guardian after their death, or when saving a respectful life is contingent upon it.

Q1285: I have expressed my wish to donate my organs after my death. I was told that I should make a will in this regard and inform my heirs. Have I the right to do so?

A: There is no harm in making use of a dead person's organs for transplantation into the bodies of other people in order to save their lives or treat their illnesses. There is no objection to writing this in one's will. This ruling, however, does not cover those parts of the body, whose removal could

45

amount to *muthlah* of the body itself, or [if] severing them would violate the dignity of the dead according to the common view. (Ibid.)

[42] Q1284: Some patients suffer from irreversible brain damage which results in the disappearance of all kinds of neurological activities associated with deep coma plus the inability to respire and respond to all motor sensory stimulations. In such cases it is not probable at all to restore these activities and the heart could only work temporarily by itself with the aid of a respirator. This condition, which is called in medicine "brain death," does not continue more than a few hours /days...On the other hand, there are other patients whose lives can only be saved by the transplantation of organs being taken from those who suffer from brain death. Is the use of organs taken from such patients for this purpose permissible?

A: If the removal of the organs from the patient described in the question would precipitate his death, it is not permissible. Otherwise, if the removal of such organs is made with his prior permission, or the use of the removed organ is the only way to save a respected life, there is no objection to it. (Ibid.)

God, the Living

Ayatollah Ja'far Subhani

The word *hayy* (living) has been used fourteen times in the Qur'an - four of which are a description of God. For example, the Qur'an says:

اَللّٰهُ لا إِلٰهَ إِلاَّ هُوَ الْحَىُّ الْقَيُّوم

God - there is no god except Him. (3:2)

وَ عَنَتِ الْوُجُوهُ لِلْحَىِّ الْقَيُّوم وَ قَد خابَ من حَمل ظُلماً

All faces shall be humbled before the Living One, the All-Sustainer, and he will fail who bears [the onus of] wrongdoing. (20:111)

وَ تَوَكَّلْ عَلَى الْحَىِّ الَّذِى لا يَمُوتُ وَ سَبِّح بِحَمْدِه...

All faces shall be humbled before the Living One, the All-Sustainer, and he will fail who bears [the onus of] wrongdoing. (25:58)

هُوَ الْحَىُّ لا إِلٰهَ إِلاَّ هُوَ فَادْعُوهُ مُخْلِصِينَ لَهُ الدِّين...

He is the Living One, there is no god except Him. So supplicate Him, putting exclusive faith in Him. All praise belongs to God, the Lord of the Worlds. (40:65)

In the verses mentioned above, God is described as *al-Hayy* (living). Now the question here is, does the word *hayāt* (life) means the same when used for Allah or other possible beings, or does it mean something different? Not only can we pose this question about the word *hayāt* (life), but we can also ask the same thing about other attributes, like *'ilm* (knowledge), *qudrah* (power) and *sam'* (hearing), as well. Some theologians refuse to investigate this topic further and say that, while we can assume that Allah is *hayy* and living, we should not research its deeper meaning. They do not see the necessity for acquiring wisdom and reason in order to understand the Islamic sciences and are satisfied with their surface appearance, yet the Qur'an encourages us to think about religious issues. Therefore, there should be no limit to our investigation within the religious sciences and we should benefit from the light of intellect to eradicate ignorance.

The natural scientists - whose subject is material being - delineate four qualities of life:

1. Digestion and excretion

2. Growth and development

3. Birth and reproduction

4. Action and reaction

However, it is obvious that these qualities do not express the true meaning of life but only show the effects of life in natural beings. Furthermore, due to the fact that they have only given one definition for all living beings, from plants to humans, they are satisfied with the four qualities that they have provided. Yet we find that, in some beings, there are qualities which are more apparent than these four, such as sensation and awareness, which refer to animal attributes, or thinking and reasoning, which is specific to human beings. Yet these attributes are not in fact the reality of life itself but refer instead to its impacts. Thus, it can even be said that the true meaning of life is incomprehensible and the only things which we can truly perceive are limited to the impacts of life.

So far we've become familiar with the meaning of life as well as the attributes of three kinds of living beings. Now we should try to understand the foundation of life and its different levels. Perhaps, after careful study, we could come up with the idea that the foundation of life lies in activity *and* sensation and that exists in all the above-mentioned living beings, albeit with different levels. It is because of the plants' response to outside stimuli that we consider them to be alive; as if the action relates to some kind of sensation that precipitated its response. Even though science has not proven the existence of sensation in all plants, we can see that, in some of them, at least, the existence of sensation is obvious. For instance, if the top part of a palm tree is cut or put in water, the tree dries out and becomes barren. When growing plants confront obstacles in their path, they change their direction. These occurrences indicate that it is possible for plants to enjoy minor types of sensation.

Animals, because they are a higher level species, benefit from a more advanced type of action and sensation. They all possess the qualities of awareness and sensation in conjunction with their actions, although the levels of these qualities might differ among various types of animals. This foundation also exists in human beings, along with greater awareness and reasoning.

According to this analysis, we could say that the foundation of life, then, includes actions coupled with awareness. However, this foundation, besides consisting of three separate levels, includes a set of normal actions that are not actually the essentials of life but rather the essentials of a lower level of life called plant life.

When we see this foundation to be so immense in a being, and thus imagine a being that is so great and limitless in knowledge and actions, then this being would literally be the All-Doer and the All-Perceiving that inevitably deserves the attribute of living and therefore should be called the Infinite Living. The life of a possible existent being that surely has a beginning and ending, depends on that of a necessary existent, while the divine life is eternal; no beginning and no ending can be imagined for it. Imam Baqir (a) says:

> Truly God, the Blessed and the High was, when nothing other than him existed, a light without any darkness, and truthful without any lie, and knowing without any ignorance, and living without death. He is like that now and will remain like that forever.[1]

Imam Kazim (a) says:

> He was living without [any specific] quality and place and He was not in anything or over anything. He was a living God without created life, rather He was living by Himself.[2]

Due to the eternality of life, and because of the fact that it is related to His essence, the Qur'an says:

> All faces shall be humbled before the Living One, the All-Sustainer, and he will fail who bears [the onus of] wrongdoing. (25:78)

---

[1] Saduq, *Al-Tawhid*, p. 141.

[2] Ibid.

Human Life

Ayatollah Misbah Yazdi

Everything in this world undergoes changes which affect its nature, including inanimate creatures. Yet even though inanimate creatures have a small area of internal growth in which they develop in comparison to living creatures, most of them do not undergo a lot of noticeable changes; and this is the reason why they are called inanimate.

Other creatures experience noticeable essential changes during their course of development. For instance, if we observe the life of a flower, we can see that it undergoes numerous changes within a matter of weeks or months. It grows new leaves and blossoms, and not long after, these leaves will be replaced with new ones. A tree also experiences different shapes and forms during its lifespan. An old tree was once a young plant, eventually growing older and stronger every day to become what it is now. In contrast, the soil in which a tree grows does not noticeably change its form, size or appearance throughout the months and years.

Another behaviour seen in plants is that they produce seeds that can be replanted in order to become plants themselves. However, this type of behaviour, or any similar behaviour, is not observed in inanimate things like soil, water, or stone, etc.

Animals also possess the same qualities seen in plants, in addition to other qualities like motion and sensation. So by a general assessment here, we can initially divide creatures into two groups: living creatures, like plants, animals, and humans, and lifeless or inanimate creatures.

The attribute of "living" is also occasionally used for a place that contains life and living creatures. The Qur'an has used the term *"reviving the earth"* to signify the growth of plants and other assorted life on a dry and dead land:

$$\text{فَأَحْيَا بِهِ الأَرْضَ مِنْ بَعْدِ مَوْتِهَا}$$

He revives the earth after its death. (29:63)

The difference between living and lifeless creatures is in fact so obvious that people most likely never engage in intellectual arguments trying to distinguish which is which. Yet examining the true meaning of life and presenting its meaning with a precise, logical answer is not an easy task. There are arguments among modern scientists, as well as those of previous generations, regarding this issue. The most important argument is between the schools of "Animism" and "Fatalism." Thus, we can ask, is life an immaterial state which cannot be formed simply by natural factors, or is life nothing but a physical phenomenon in which physical rules and explanations will suffice? Is the thing which we refer to as "spirit," "soul," or "mind" physical in character or is it something which is beyond the physical?

As far as the scope of this article goes, mentioning the theories of different philosophers, and extrapolating upon them, is not our concern here. So let us continue discussing different forms of life, and proceed to the main point of this article, which is human life.

Life, from what can be generally observed, has two forms or levels: the kind of life that exists in plants, and has the attribute of growth and reproduction, and the kind that exists in animals, which also has the attribute of motion and sensation, in addition to growth and reproduction. Human life is also a type of animal life. It has all the aforementioned attributes, and when it loses these qualities, it is no longer considered to be alive.

Obviously, life, as we can see from the points above, has the same components in all animals. But considered more carefully, the term "humanity" depends on human beings possessing something more than animals, which is specific only to them. Therefore, human life is superior to animal life because of this finer quality or attribute which it possesses. So when we say that "humanity" is a quality which is specific to humans that distinguishes between human and animal life, we are naturally led to believe that when this quality is lost in human beings, even if they still have the qualities seen in animal life, "human life" has ceased to exist.

The distinction between human beings and other animals can be discussed under two different categories - namely, their ranks and their true nature. The differences which are related to their ranks refer to the fact that humans are superior to other animals in certain biological dimensions. In other words, human beings are animals which are more perfect than other animals. However, such superiorities cannot be counted as the fundamental superiorities of human beings. The actual superiority of a human being lies in the specific reality that he is able to ascertain and which animals completely lack. Human beings potentially have this reality by birth, and, by following the teachings of prophets and holy people, they can get close to the actualization of this reality. Finally, it is the grace of God that gives them the light of human life.

اومن كان ميتآ فاحييناه و جعلنا له نورا يمشى به فى الناس

Is he who was lifeless, then we gave him life and provided him with a light, by which he walks among people. (6:22)

53

يا ايها الذين آمنوا استجيبوا الله و للرسول اذا دعاكم لما
يحييكم

O you who have faith. Answer God and the
Apostle when he summons you to that which will
give you life. (8:24)

Man, once he has achieved this life, possesses a different type of
vision and a different type of hearing than other people because
those who lack this level of life are blind and deaf from the point
of view of human life.

من كان فى هذه اعمى فهو فى الاخره اعمى و اضل
سبيلا

But whoever has been blind in this [world], will be
blind in the Hereafter and [even] more astray from
the [right] way. (17:72)

لهم قلوب لا يفقهون بها ولهم اعين لا يبصرون بها
ولهم ءاذان لا يسمعون بها اولئك كالانعام بل هم اضل
اولئك هم الغافلون

They have hearts with which they do not
understand, they have eyes with which they do not
see, they have ears with which they do not hear;
they are like cattle rather they are more astray. It is
they who are the heedless. (7:179)

Just as animal and plant life have an origin, referred to as *the
plant spirit* and *the animal spirit*, human life also has an origin
which has different levels and names. In religious texts, this
origin is most often referred to as *the spirit of faith* (*ruh al-imān*).
In some hurried (*mursal*) traditions, one of its levels is called the
nātiqah qudsiyyah, while its highest level is called *kulliyyah
ilāhiyyah.*

Zurarah narrates: Once I asked Imam Sadiq, "Please explain to me the Prophet's saying: 'The fornicator does not commit fornication in the state of faith (*imān*).' He replied, "In that time, the spirit of faith leaves him." I asked for an explanation of the spirit of faith. Imam replied: "It is a being that you can understand in this way. Have you experienced times when you attempt to commit a bad deed and an internal reality stops you?" I said: "Yes." Imam continued: "That is the spirit of faith."

Aban ibn Taghlib, one of the great students of Imam Sadiq (a), narrates that that the Imam once said: "The spirit of faith is one and has come from God. It has been distributed among different people. Through it they have affection and companionship among themselves and it will leave them again as a single unity and go back to Him."

Human life, once it has become fully developed, joins the eternal life; a life which, compared with temporary earthly life, will make earthly life look like death, unlike what materialists imagine. The Holy Qur'an says:

وَ ما هذِهِ الْحَياةُ الدُّنْيا إِلاَّ لَهْوٌ وَ لَعِبٌ وَ إِنَّ الدَّارَ الْآخِرَةَ لَهِيَ الْحَيَوانُ لَوْ كانُوا يَعْلَمُونَ

The life of this world is nothing but diversion and play. But the abode of the Hereafter is indeed life, had they known! (29:64)

The Holy Qur'an also relates that the sinners on Judgment Day will say:

يا ليتنى قدمت لحياتى

He will say, 'Alas, had I sent for my life.' (89:24)

Reaching that level of life is not limited only to the period after death. Some people may turn their backs on the material world and turn towards the spiritual world before they die. Describing

55

those who have revived their hearts by the remembrance of God, Imam Ali (a) says:

فكانما قطعوا الدنيا الي الاخره و هم فيها فشاهدوا ماوراء ذلك فكانما اطلعوا غيوب اهل البرزخ في طول الاقامه فيه و حققت القيامه عليهم عداتها ، فكشفوا غطاء ذلك لاهل الدنيا حتي كانهم يرون ما لا يري الناس و يسمعون ما لا يسمعون

It is as though they have finished the journey of this world towards the next world and have beheld what lies beyond it. Consequently, they have become acquainted with all that befell them in the interstice during their long stay therein, and the Day of Judgement fulfils its promises for them. Therefore, they removed the curtain from these things for the people of the world, till it was as though they were seeing what people did not see and were hearing what people did not hear. (*Nahj al-Balaghah*, Sermon 220)

Indeed, it can be understood from the verse (17:72) that was mentioned earlier, that anyone missing this reality in this life and has not opened his heart and mind to the eternal truth in this world, will also miss it in the life Hereafter. This can also be argued philosophically.

The Fundamentality of the Soul

Ayatollah Mutahhari

The problem of body and soul has always been a dynamic and controversial issue. It has been discussed in a variety of ways, by different people, in various times, and this has somehow changed the character of the general concept. Most of the scientific issues are only discussed by experts; however, everyone has talked about the issue of the soul throughout history. For an issue with such importance, these discussions by non-experts can be harmful, since their arguments shape its general concept, thus making it appear different from what it actually is. This then complicates the task for students and researchers, and even causes confusion on occasion.

This is one of the issues that, at some point in our lives, we have all pondered, shaped our ideas about, and finally solved according to our own perceptions and thinking. Everyone finds answers to these kinds of questions in some manner. Of course, this does not happen by chance. One of the first questions which the curious nature of man might ask is: What am I and what is this universe in which I live? Inevitably, man has to satisfy himself with answers to these questions, and therefore everyone will attain some sort of self-knowledge and develop a personal worldview.

Thus, the issue of body and soul is one of those controversial issues for which almost everyone has an opinion. Everyone has heard a lot about this topic since childhood - from parents, teachers, speakers - and later, by reading about the subject in books and articles. Therefore, a considerable number of people, after seeing the title of this article, might suppose that they are going to be told that the soul is a mysterious being which has been hidden in the body for certain reasons, that it acts more irregularly than jinns and beasts, and that the body is nothing but an outer layer for the soul that is responsible for all the actions which a person performs.

Indeed, many people may be ready to hear these statements. One might even be reminded of what he has read in poetry - that the soul is a heavenly creature which has been imprisoned within the body...We are not trying to criticize the language of poetry here. Poetry is meant to be like this. However, the language of philosophy obviously cannot be the same as poetry. Their differing goals require different methods and objectives. Thus, the kind of language and logic used in every subject must suit its particular needs. Accordingly, we can find people who have written different types of works, like poetry and philosophy, have used different languages about the very same subject. Their language of philosophy is different from that of poetry. One particular instance of this difference is in Avicenna's approach to the subject of body and soul in his two philosophical books, *Al-Shifā* and *Al-Ishārāt va al-Tanbihāt* with that of his famous poem, *'Ayniyyah*.

Hence, we have to distinguish between the language of science and philosophy from that of poets and orators, so that we do not make the same mistakes the materialists have made. In fact, even amongst philosophers, sometimes we find theories which are similar to the theories of poets. The famous theory of Plato is a good example, which states that the soul pre-exists the body and that when the body is made ready the soul descends and dwells in the body. Plato's theory of soul can be considered to be an instance of body and soul dualism, since he finds each object to be two separate things whose relation is like that of a bird to its nest. However, it was not long before Plato's theory was questioned by his student, Aristotle.

Aristotle realized that the relation of the soul to the body cannot be underestimated nor can it be considered to be the same as the relation of a bird to its nest or a rider to his ride. The relationship, certainly, must be a deeper and a more natural one. Aristotle was the first philosopher to view the relation of the soul to the body as the relation of form to matter, with the exception that the rational faculty, due to its immaterialness, is not considered to be form within matter, but rather form that exists *along with* matter. Hence, in Aristotle's philosophical theories, there is no trace of the soul being an eternal and fully actualized substance; the soul is created. The soul merely consists of potentiality and capability in the beginning and has no knowledge in advance. It actualises all its potential knowledge in this world. The theory of Avicenna reflects the same kind of approach, with a slight difference. It can be seen that, in the theories of Aristotle and Avicenna, the dualism between soul and body, which is observable in the theory of Plato, is reduced to a great extent, and that the basis for both theories is Aristotle's famous theories of "matter and form" and "generation and corruption" (*al-kawn wa'l-fasād*).

This theory had advantages over the Platonic theory. It deserves consideration since, instead of the dualism of the soul and the body, it sees a kind of real and substantial unity between them. However, this theory has its own problems and ambiguities. Its most important problems lie in the manner of clarifying the natural relation between matter and form and in explaining the issue of generation and corruption.

Therefore, more steps needed to be taken in the world of science and philosophy if man is to ever uncover this mystery or at least gain a reasonable idea of the concept. Now let us see how initial steps were taken.

Indeed, the very first step was taken when Europe became ready for a revolution. After the revolution, nothing was immune from change, regardless of its position in science or intellectual thought. New ideas and theories were established for almost every issue, including the problem of body and soul. René Descartes, the famous French philosopher, established a new kind of body-soul dualism, which later drew the attention of scholars to approve, disapprove, or reform the theory.[1]

Descartes' thoughts led him to believe in the reality of three things: God, soul and body. Considering the soul to be a thinking substance with no dimension, and the body as a dimensional substance with no intellect and rationality, he distinguished between body and soul.

His theory was first questioned by European philosophers who rightly claimed that Descartes had only taken one aspect into consideration, which was the difference of the body and soul. They believed that he had not provided any explanation about the relation of the body to the soul and wondered how these two substances - that he believed were completely separated - could join with each other. The important point about the problem of body and soul is how to explain their relation and their unity.

Indeed, Descartes' theory was a return to the old theory of Plato, reminding us of the old bird-nest relation. Since Descartes believed in innate and inherent knowledge from the beginning, in some points, he knows soul to be actual,[1] thus his theory was close to the theory of Plato. Furthermore, similar to Plato's theory, Descartes' theory falls short in explaining the relation of body to soul.

The issue of the relation of soul and body was so important that scholars could not accept for this question to be neglected in any theory. They were not satisfied by simply explaining the dualism and divergence of body and soul. Therefore, all efforts by intelligent scholars after Descartes attempted to discover and explain the relation between them.

One who has a general understanding of philosophical studies in the contemporary age will know how much effort recent philosophers have put into finding the relation between the physical and spiritual affairs of human beings. Many schools of thought have been developed which exaggerate various parts of the issue to the extent that some people have come to believe that spiritual affairs are a natural part of material substances, thus leaving out any kind of dualism between the soul and the body. Some have viewed the body and other material substances as unreal and simply a showcase for the soul to omit the dualism of the soul and the body. Tiring of the strenuous efforts required to resolve this matter, some scholars have found this issue to be beyond human understanding.

Despite the arguments of recent philosophers not proceeding very far on the essence of spiritual affairs and the quality of the soul-body relationship, the tireless work of other scientists, especially in the fields of biology and, more importantly, physiology and psychology, achieved great results. While it is possible that these scientists were not concerned with the characteristics of spiritual affairs and how the soul relates to the body, their work has certainly paved the ground for research in this field, which will be mentioned later.

Earlier in this article, we mentioned the theory of Aristotle and Avicenna and pointed out that the emphasis on body-soul dualism has been lessened and more stress has been put on their aspects relating to unity. This is due to the famous hypothesis of Aristotle, the theory of forms and matter.

Now we are going to review how this issue was treated by Islamic philosophers after Avicenna.

After Avicenna, no new research was done directly on this issue by Islamic philosophers. However, Islamic philosophers made massive improvements within the most common and fundamental issues of primary philosophy, those relating to existence.[2] These improvements had an indirect but important impact on most of the philosophical issues, including the issue of motion and the issues of the dualism/monism of the body and the soul.

Since there is no room for going into detail on this subject, we shall only call attention to some key points. Mulla Sadra, who was the pioneer of the scientific revolution in the issues of existence, concluded from the new rules he had established that, in addition to the apparent and transverse motion which can be seen in the world, there is also a deep and substantial motion that goes on in the substance of the world. It is this substantial motion that is the origin of apparent and tangible motions. If we are to imagine matter and form, it has to be through this motion. The formation and consistency of physical types is based on the law of motion, not on generation and corruption.

The soul is also an outcome of the law of motion. The origin of the soul's existence is physical - matter has the ability to create something supernatural within itself and there are no walls between the physical and the supernatural world. There are no obstacles that a material being could not, in its levels of progress and perfection, turn into an immaterial being. Platonic ideas about the origins of the soul are completely wrong, as are Aristotle's; the kind of relation between matter and life and soul and body are more natural and more substantial than what they have supposed. This relation is like the relation between the strong and perfect level of a substance with its weak and imperfect one. In other words, the relation between soul and body is like the relation of one dimension with other dimensions. That is, matter, in its progress and perfection, in addition to the three material dimensions, and the dimension of time, which is the amount of essential and substantial motion, expands in another dimension. This dimension is independent of the other four which are related to time and place. Of course, by referring to it as a dimension, we do not mean that it is similar to a continuous quantity and that, like other quantities, can be divided into parts in the mind. Rather, by referencing dimension, we mean only to point out that matter finds a new aspect and develops and expands in another direction, reaching a level where it will lose all its material qualities.

This introduction was to show us that, before having a true understanding of the body-soul relationship, any effort to discuss whether the soul is fundamental or not, and whether it is a result of the combination of matter's parts or not, will be in vain. However, after this issue has become clear, we can then discuss whether the spiritual qualities are a result of the combination of material parts, like all other properties that matter possesses solely or in combination, or if matter does not possess these qualities, as long as it is in its material state and these qualities appear when matter develops in its essence, and achieves a level of existence in which it will be non-material and non-physical, and the spiritual qualities we mentioned are a result of this level of existence and reality.

At this level, we do not need to limit our discussion to the human soul and man's spiritual affairs. Rather, we can continue our discussion in the affairs and effects of life in its entirety.

The difference between the mental and other effects of life is about abstractness and non-abstractness, which we will not discuss at this point. What is more important at this juncture is to discuss how the soul is not the quality and effect of matter. It is a substantial perfection found by matter, that when found, produces more various effects than the effects of matter. Of course, this is not related only to the human or animal soul; it includes all living beings and all kinds of life.

Whatever the reality of life is, whether it is understandable by human beings or not, this much is for sure: some beings that we consider to be living creatures, i.e., plants and animals, have certain types of actions and qualities that are not observed in other beings that are inanimate and lifeless.

These beings have the quality of self-protection. They protect themselves against environmental factors. That is, living creatures prepare themselves for living in an environment with an entirely inner power, organizing the tools within themselves in a way in which they can fight against environmental factors to their advantage and use them to stay alive.

All living things have the quality of adapting to the environment, which originates from an inner activity. On the contrary, non-living things do not possess this quality, which means if a non-living thing is put into an environment where all conditions are in the direction of its destruction, it will do nothing to survive.

For instance, living things can get used to new things. When a living being is annoyed by an external factor, at first it will be affected and disturbed and will lose its balance. However, little by little, it will get used to the external factor and form a kind of immunity against it. This immunity is due to the quality of adapting to the environment and is achieved as much as conditions allow. If a plant, the body of an animal or an organ of the body is in an inappropriate environment, where its life and balance are threatened, it will gradually equip itself so that it can easily resist the threat. Human hands are so soft and smooth that when they first have to haul a hard and heavy material, they cannot tolerate it. However, the same hands will gradually get used to this activity. An internal force changes their tissues accordingly, so that they can withstand the external factor.

Living creatures perform the activity of feeding. Automatically, affected by an internal factor, they absorb outside materials, decompose them and use their particular combinations for survival. This feature does not exist in inanimate creatures.

If we look around, we will see that living creatures, no matter where they live, grow gradually and become complete. They increase their power to the point where they can reproduce, then they die and continue life through the survival of their offspring.

Life, wherever it exists, influences the environment and overcomes lifeless elements of nature, changing their form and combinations. Life is the sketch-maker, the designer and the engineer. It has the ability to progress and achieve perfection, it has a goal and it is selective. Life knows its direction and its destination. Life moves gently towards the destination that it chose million years ago. Its specific destination is not possibly anything other than perfection in its greatest degree.

These qualities appear in living creatures and do not exist in lifeless creatures. As Cressy Morrison has said, matter does not contain initiative on its own and it is only life that constantly manifests new and original forms and designs.

Thus we can clearly understand that life on its own is a special force, a separate perfection and an additional actuality that comes into existence in matter, and brings forth different and additional activities.

We mentioned previously that the research of European scientists has resulted in significant information in the field of biology that has paved the way for the philosophical consideration of the problem of the body and the soul, though this may have not been the intention of those scientists themselves.

Indeed, significant research has been done on the issue of life which makes the originality of the life force obvious. A great number of scientists have noticed this and accepted the originality of the life force. They believe that the life force is a force that is added to matter in its natural process and the effects of life are all due to this force, and not to the combination or division of the parts of matter. Combination and division are a necessary process in the appearance of life but is not enough. Furthermore, when we closely examine the theories of those who have denied the originality of the life force, such as Lamarck, and who have stated that living nature should only be examined physically, we understand that the reason that has impelled them to deny the fundamentality of the life force is that they thought this would be equal to an existential dualism between *the life force* and *matter and its effects*. They thought if the life force was to be original, it has to be independent from the environment and its elements, must be the same in every environment, cannot be affected by environmental elements and cannot be dependent on the physical and chemical activities of the body. However, scientific studies prove these theories to be wrong. Lamarck says life is not more than a physical state; all qualities of life have a physical or chemical reason and their source lies in the body of living matter.

It seems as if Lamarck has supposed that, if the life force is to be original, it has to be independent from physical and chemical reasons and its source should not be in the body of the creature.

As we said, Descartes' theory of dualism, which was a return to the old Platonic idea of dualism, did much harm, since it made the scientists refuse to see the substantial relation of life to the body whenever they thought about the fundamentality of the life force, and thus they always thought in two different directions. Descartes chose the dualism of the body (whose property is dimensional) and the soul (whose property is thinking and sensation) in order to approach this issue, therefore, he found them too distant from each other.

Thus he had to deny life as a fundamental force in other creatures. It is a wonder that he considered the structure of animals - excluding man - to be only mechanical and denied any kind of perception or sense existing within them. He claimed that animals have no perception or emotion. They do not feel pleasure or pain and that what we can perceive of their behaviour, whether moving in a certain situation or singing, is not a result of their having perception or sense. Rather it is only that these mechanical structures have been created to perform such acts in certain situations, giving us the delusion of thinking that they have will and sensation.

In any case, the theory of the fundamentality of the life force has been completely confirmed by recent scientific investigations. The theory of evolution, too, was a proof for the originality of the life force and its dominance over matter and non-living nature. Darwin, who developed the theory of evolution, not only did not have the intention to prove the originality of the life force, but also based his theory, at first, on natural selection and deemed natural selection to be the result of random and purposeless changes. However, in the end, when he became aware of the mystery of development and the secret of the regular process of species evolution, he found himself helplessly accepting a kind of personality for living nature. Darwin did not intend to examine the life force, yet he achieved this conclusion automatically through his studies. This fact was so obvious in his statements that some researchers told him that he spoke of natural selection as an active force and a supernatural power.[3]

Those who studied the psychological aspects of human beings discovered the same results, also without trying to look for the fundamentality of human life or being concerned about the philosophical outcomes of their research. Freud, who founded the psychoanalytic school of psychiatry, revolutionised the field of psychology. In his studies, he realized that the works of physiologists, who focused on examining the brain, were not enough for curing mental illnesses. He discovered a hidden system of awareness in which the natural awareness of human beings is comparably very shallow: the unconscious.

Freud understood that the mental effects derived from psychological complexes can also cause and lead to various illnesses. Hence, while trying to help cure patients, the analyst should use mental approaches so that the patient can resolve repressed conflicts and recover, and then even the physical symptoms of his or her illness would also disappear.

Curing mental illnesses - and even some physical illnesses - through mental and emotional approaches is not a new discovery, since physicians such as Muhammad ibn Zakariyā Rāzī and Avicenna used the same methodology centuries ago. But today, this field has greatly expanded and some of its methods are extraordinary; they confirm the fundamentality of life, especially the fundamentality of the soul in human beings. The interesting point in Freudianism was the discovery of the unconscious and the role of a series of psychological complexes. Moral and psychological illnesses were previously thought to be habits. A habit is a state formed by the repetition of a certain act and is known to be a physical process. It is similar to when we bend a straight stick and it returns to its original state. If we bend it again, it will return once more, however, it will be less than the first time. If we continue to bend the stick several times, the stick will remain bent. It is said that habits are similar to when a stick remains bent or a paper remains folded. The repetition of an act leaves permanent effects on the brain that are called either virtue or vice. However, the theory of the unconscious and the theory of complexes prove that moral processes are independent of the mentioned processes.

Freud did not want to prove the originality of the life force in his theory, nor did he want to prove the dominance of life upon matter; when he moved from his scientific studies, in which he has shown great proficiency, to the realm of philosophical reasoning, a subject in which he was not qualified, he constructed theories which were not suitable to his status. Despite this, however, his scientific studies are admirable.

Some of Freud's students, such as Carl Jung, took a different direction in the way they used psychological theories for philosophical reasoning, and to a large extent, clarified the aspect of the fundamentality of the life force in these theories, giving Freud's premise a supernatural aspect.

As we mentioned earlier, the main problem regarding this issue is not about finding the differences between matter and life, or the body and life, since even before the obvious clues and proofs were found by European researchers concerning the fundamentality of the life force, simple observations provided enough support for this fact. Yet the main problem here lies in the manner of clarifying the relation between matter and life. The drawbacks of this issue caused a lot of scientists to refuse to believe in the fundamentality of the life force, yet as we mentioned before, this problem was best solved in the philosophy of Mulla Sadra.

The fundamentality of the life force does have a supernatural aspect. If life was an effect of matter, it would not have any kind of supernatural aspect since it would be a hidden effect within combined or divided matter. It also means that when a living being is born, nothing is created and no development can be found within matter. However, according to the theory of the fundamentality of the life force, matter lacks life in its very nature and thus life is created and granted when matter becomes potential and ready for receiving it. In other words, in its motion and development towards perfection, matter becomes alive. It finds a perfection which it had previously lacked and possesses new effects and features it did not previously have. Thus, a being is really created when it is born.

A question may arise here that matter, while in separation, does not have living features. What is wrong, then, with saying that the composition and interactions of components within matter are the cause of living features? The answer is as follows: when material or non-material components are mixed and subsequently interact with each other, each one of them imparts some of it features to the others and in turn receives some of theirs. Thus, it is impossible that a mixture of components with certain features results in the creation of a feature that is not composed of the overall features of the components involved, unless the combination of these components, prepares the ground for the emergence of a power greater than the power of each component involved, and that power is created as a substantial quality, giving the components a real unity. Therefore, the question - what if, due to a combination of matters, the components of the matters acquire a living quality through their combination - needs clarification. The question is reasonable if what is meant is the providing of a new condition and potential for the emergence of the fundamental life force through the interaction between the different components of matter. But if what is meant here is the emergence of a living quality without its former presence, through the combination of matters which do not possess that quality, we must answer that it is not possible.

Yet another option remains and, therefore, it may be asked as follows: it is true that matter is essentially lifeless and that life is a power which is superior to the powers of lifeless matter. But just as the amount of energy in lifeless creatures is fixed, and their creation and elimination is simply transmission of energy from one part to another, we can assume that there is a kind of special energy for life, so that the forces of life, similar to other forces, are neither created nor made. Rather as a result of certain additions and subtractions and transfer of energies, they move from one place to another. Therefore, becoming alive is not an act of creation, but rather the transformation of life energy and life force.

In response, we must first of all say that the concept of life energy has to be explained. Is this energy dead and non-living in its nature or is it living and alive? And if, according to the second assumption, it is indeed alive, is its life something which is independent of its nature that has been mixed with it, or there is a third assumption i.e. life is its nature? According to the first and the second assumption, there is no difference between this energy and other energies in terms of being the life force or of causing life. Since this energy is either non-living (according to the first assumption), or the life force is something out of its nature that is added to it. Therefore, this energy cannot be the source of life that we look for. Only a third possibility remains, which means that an abstract being (the life energy) descends and becomes corporeal while at the same time preserving its features. This is impossible.[4]

Secondly, suppose that we deny the theory of creation in non-living matter and accept that the emergence of beings is due to nothing but the combination and division of matter's components and the transmission of energy. However, according to what scientists believe, this cannot be true in the case of living creatures. Life cannot be thought of as something that possesses a permanent amount within the world. The coming to life of creatures cannot be justified as the transmission of life from one point to another or, in fact, as some kind of reincarnation. Life does not have a certain and permanent amount; indeed, it has been increasing since the day it emerged on earth, and if some amount of it is destroyed at a certain point, say, when a few creatures die somewhere on earth, this power then does not appear somewhere else. Of course, life and death are a kind of expanding and decreasing, but only of the kind that is supplied from a state of being which is superior to the universe. When life is given, the soul is unwrapped and enters the body and when life is taken, it is removed from the body. Life is a blessing that comes from the unseen and returns to it.

Here, in order to support the above statement, we mention the viewpoint of Oswald Culpe in criticizing materialism, from his book, *An Introduction to Philosophy*. He believes that materialism is in contradiction to one of the fundamental laws of physics - the conservation of energy. According to this law, the amount of energy in the universe is permanent and the changes occurring around us are nothing more than the transmission of energy from one point to another and its transformation from one form to another. Based on this law, it is obvious that physical phenomena form a closed circle, and within this circle, no room can remain for other kind of phenomena, namely, mental phenomena.

Therefore, despite their complexity, rational operations are all affairs that follow the rule of cause and effect. And all the changes made to the brain by exterior causes are purely physical and chemical and are spread by the same state. This general theory neglects the rational aspect of things, since we cannot imagine the physical and material roots for mental phenomenon without any reduction in the physical energy of physical phenomenon. The only logical solution is to believe in a special kind of energy for rational operations, in addition to other chemical, electrical, thermal and mechanical energies. We also have to accept that there is a stable relation between this special energy and other energies; the kind of relation that other energies have between each other. However, none of the materialist scholars have mentioned this idea and there is no mention of this issue in their books. Furthermore, there are general criticisms of this idea that leave no chance for it to be proposed. The core of all criticisms made regarding this idea is that there is no way one can tie rational and mental operations and phenomenon to the concept of energy that the scholars of physics have defined.

As Cressy Morrison says in his book:

> The appearance of intellectual man is too complicated to be considered as changes in matter and to neglect the role of a creator, and if we do not see it that way, then man will be a mechanical tool that another hand is making work. Now, let's see who is the one that is making this machine function. So far, science has not been able to explain nor understand this operator, but the fact that the nature of this operator is not of material combinations is obvious.

He also believes that:

> Matter only acts according to the rules and the systems it belongs to; atoms and particles are subject to the laws related to gravity, chemical interactions, and atmospheric and electrical effects. Matter is not creative, and it is only life that, at every moment, creates new forms and novel beings.

When philosophers discuss the cause and effect issue or the unknown phenomena of nature, they talk about spiritual effects and power (e.g. Avicenna in the tenth chapter of his book, *al-Ishārāt*). Mulla Sadra, while speaking about the cause and effect theory in his book *al-Asfār*, has written a chapter called "About How Thought and Imagination Sometimes Cause Some Things to Happen." His intention in this chapter is to show the dominance and effect of thought and imagination, which are two of life's affairs, on matter. One of the things he mentions in this chapter is the effect of inculcation and the delusion of sickness or wellness in causing sickness or wellness.

Now, to avoid expanding the article further, we will not discuss this subject and a lot of other related subjects.[5] It will suffice to say that, today, there is no longer any room for Democritusian ideas that the universe is nothing but a mechanical system and creation is nothing but a composition of atoms. Scientific research has proved all the materialists wrong. No more can one say, like Descartes, that if I was given matter and motion, I would have created the universe. The universe is too complicated to be limited to matter and sensible and accidental motion.

---

[1] For further information in this regard please refer to *Usul-e Falsafeh wa Rawesh-e Realism,* vol. 2.

[2] For further information and the historical order of the mentioned issues, please refer to *Usul-e Falsafeh wa Rawesh-e Realism,* vol 3.

[3] Behzad, Mahmoud, *Darwinism,* 5th edition, p. 99.

[44] It has to be noted that what philosophers mean by descendant when they claim that nature and matter are descended forms of the supernatural is a different subject and is not the same as the transformation of energy.

[5] Refer to the books on inculcation and its effects like: *Tadāwi Ruhi* by Kazim Zadeh, Iranshahr.

The Qur'an and Life

Ayatollah Mutahhari

In the previous paper, we have discussed the issue of life and soul from a philosophical perspective. We tried to understand whether the soul is a property or an effect of matter, or if matter lacks life in its nature and life is a reality on its own with certain features, and, unless life joins matter, features and effects of life cannot be found in matter. Since this was a philosophical perspective, we approached the subject philosophically. In what follows, we will discuss the topic of life from a Qur'anic perspective and discover what the Qur'an says about life, especially its relation to the supernatural world and God's will.

The term "life" has been mentioned many times in the Qur'an. In many verses, God speaks of things becoming alive, living beings' consecutive coming into existence, life's progress, the order of creation of living beings, and the effects of life (i.e. intelligence, reason, cognition, hearing, vision, guidance, inspiration, instinct, etc.) as the signs of God's wisdom and design. While each of these can be an interesting issue on its own, we are not going to discuss these points for now. One of the life-related issues pointed out in the Holy Qur'an is that life is in God's hands, it is He who gives life, and He who takes it away. By mentioning this, the Holy Qur'an actually states that life is not under the control of anyone other than God. No one other than Him can give or take life. This is the subject which we are going to discuss now.

In *Surah al-Baqarah*, Prophet Abraham is quoted as saying to the oppressor of his time:

ربى الذى يحيى و يميت

My Lord is He who gives life and brings death.
(2:258)

In *Surah al-Mulk,* God is described in this way:

الذى خلق الموت و الحياه

He who created death and life... (67:2)

There are a lot of verses in the Qur'an that introduce God as the only one who "gives life" and "brings death" and relate these actions directly to Him. That is, those verses leave out the mention of anyone other than Him. Also, the verses which point out the reviving of the dead by some prophets specifically mention that this can only be done with the permission of God. For instance, the Qur'an says:

و رسولا الى بنى اسرائيل انى قد جئتكم بايه من ربكم انى اخلق لكم من الطين كهيئة الطير فانفخ فيه فيكون طيرا باذن الله و ابرى ء الاكمه و الابرص و احيى الموتى باذن الله

And [he will be] an apostle to the Children of Israel, [and he will declare] 'I have certainly brought you a sign from your Lord. I will create for you the form of a bird out of clay, then I will breathe into it, and it will become a bird by God's leave. And I heal the blind and the leper and I revive the dead by God's leave... (3:49)

Overall, the main difference between the materialists and monotheist scholars is that monotheists believe that the root, origin and creator of life is beyond matter, but materialists

76

believe that matter itself is the creator. Yet the way the Qur'an points us to the fact that God is the Creator of life, rather than anyone else, differs from the monotheist's scholars point of view. The difference might seem to be small but it is of great importance. In fact, the way the Qur'an points out this issue can be counted among one of the signs which prove that the Qur'an is a miracle. If the monotheist scholars understand the Qur'anic approach to this issue, they will be able to solve it for themselves, and then convince and guide the materialists and remove their ignorance.

Normally, when scholars want to relate life to God's will and unity, they start from the dawn of life and ask how life initially came into existence. Certain scientific proofs show that there is indeed a beginning for the appearance of life on earth. In other words, none of the living beings, including plants, animals and humans, have been here forever, since earth itself has a limited and specific age. Furthermore, earth, in its estimated millions of years of existence, has not always been capable of containing living organisms.

So, how did these creatures first appear?

Based on what we are able to observe, each creature is born from another creature of its own type; a wheat plant is created from a wheat seed which is again created by another wheat plant. Similarly, a horse is born from another horse and a human being from another human being. There can never be a plant or animal created from a mass of soil; the origin of a living creature's existence is another living creature that reproduces via egg, sperm or other means.

Now, a question arises: how has this been accomplished in the first place? Does each kind of creature have a specific first ancestor? If that is true, how has that first ancestor appeared? As we said earlier, a living creature is only created by another living creature and it cannot simply appear from nowhere. So inevitably there must have been some kind of exception or miracle which happened, and this creation must have been done by God.

We can make another assumption in which all creatures derive from one origin and are siblings of each other. In this case, too, the question is raised again that, supposing all the species are rooted in one origin and the origin of all organisms has been unicellular, now where has that first unicellular organism come from? Has science not proved that organisms can only be brought to life through another organism? So, then, is the first organism an exception to this rule? Is it a miracle made by God?[1]

At this point, materialists inevitably offer theories which do not even convince themselves. On the contrary, monotheist scholars take this as a proof of God's existence and say that the first organism has undoubtedly come into existence through a supernatural cause - God's will. While explaining evolution and how different organisms evolved from their ancestors, Darwin, who believed in God, was left with the conundrum of the first organisms who did not have any parents. At which point, he said: They must have been created by a divine power.

In his book, *The Mystery of Man's Creation*, Cressy Morrison talks about this issue. Some say the *gemma* of life escaped from one of the planets, and, after wandering in space for many centuries, landed on planet earth. This idea is untenable since it is impossible for the *gemma* of life to survive the absolute coldness of space. And supposing it could, the cosmic rays which are spread out in space would destroy it. And again, if it passes this level, and if it should accidentally land somewhere with very good conditions for its survival, like the depth of the seas, which have several kinds of living conditions, that make for a suitable living environment. After all these issues, the question is raised, "What was the origin of that life and how did it appear on other planets?"

It is proven today that the environment - regardless of how optimal it is for life - cannot produce life. Nor can the *gemma* of life be produced with any chemical compound. The issue of life still remains an unsolved scientific problem.

Some say a very small particle of a substance, which is not observable by microscope, gathers with the many particles of the atom, disturbing their equilibrium, and forming life with the addition and subtraction of their parts. However, no one has ever claimed to have created life with any interaction between substances.

By saying this, Cressy Morrison means to prove that an intelligent creator has created and started life, for it cannot be explained by natural and material causes. Regarding the beginning of man's creation and the great change that led to the creation of a being that had reason and intellect and a force that could invent sciences, he says the appearance of the intellectual human being is too complicated to be considered as a result of changes in matter and we cannot neglect the role of a creator.

This was a sample of these groups' beliefs regarding life and its relation to God's will. It does not seem necessary to mention the words of others, since there is not much difference between their theories and what we have already mentioned.

So far man has not been able to create a living organism in laboratories. For example, he has not been able to create artificial wheat that has the features of real wheat, such as being able to grow and seed when planted. Neither has he been able to create animal or human sperm that can become a real animal or human. However, scientists have not been discouraged and are still trying hard to achieve this level of knowledge. They are not certain at this time whether this goal is achievable or if it is beyond man's scientific and industrial power.

Similar to the issue of life's beginning, this future related issue, is also controversial. As expected, the monotheist scholars who believe life is in God's hands, and their view towards the relation between life and God's will is what was mentioned before, say that the effort of man to create life is pointless because the control of life is not in human hands, but is due to God alone. A human being cannot create life by his will using scientific tools whenever he desires. The prophets that used to give life to a lifeless matter did so with the permission of God, and it is impossible to do such a thing without His permission. If someone does so with the permission of God, he has to be a prophet performing a miracle. And God creates miracles only through His friends and prophets.

They have taken the present inability of humans to create life as a reason for their claim. They say even now that man is capable of making wheat which has the same compound of real wheat, yet the wheat he makes is lifeless. Because life depends on God's will and His permission is definitely needed in order to give life to something, and He does not give this permission to anyone other than His prophets.

We have mentioned that the Qur'an explicitly says only God can give life and denies the interference of anything other than God in the act of creation. However, the Qur'an never tries to prove this fact by speaking about the beginning of the life of man or any other organism. Rather, it uses the current order of the universe as its witness and understands that the current system of the universe is the system of creation and formation. The Qur'an states that life is due solely to God and He is the creator of life. But when the Qur'an wants to declare that God has created life, it does not talk about the first day of life, nor does it distinguish between the first day and the other ones. The Qur'an says that the current regular developments of life are the developments of creation. For example, the Qur'an states:

و لقد خلقنا الانسان من سلالة من طين ثم جعلناه نطفة فى قرار مكين ثم خلقنا النطفة علقة فخلقنا العلقة مضغة فخلقنا المضغة عظاما فكسونا العظام لحما ثم انشأناه خلقا آخر فتبارك الله احسن الخالقين

80

Certainly We created man from an extract of clay. Then We made him a drop of [seminal] fluid [lodged] in a secure abode. Then We created the drop of fluid as a clinging mass. Then We created the clinging mass as a fleshy tissue. Then We created the fleshy tissue as bones. Then We clothed the bones with flesh. Then We produced him as [yet] another creature. So blessed is God, the best of creators. (23:12-14)

This verse mentions the development and change of a fetus through a certain system and regards these developments as consecutive stages and developments of creation.

ما لكم لا ترجون لله وقارا و قد خلقكم اطوارا

What is the matter with you that you do not look upon God with veneration, while He created you in [various] stages? (71:13-14)

يخلقكم فى بطون امهاتكم خلقا من بعد خلق فى ظلمات ثلث

He creates you in the wombs of your mothers, creation after creation, in a three-fold darkness. (39:6)

كيف تكفرون بالله و كنتم امواتا فاحياكم ثم يميتكم ثم يحييكم ثم اليه ترجعون

How can you be unfaithful to God, [seeing that] you were lifeless and He gave you life, then He will make you die, and then He shall bring you to life, and then you will be brought back to Him?" (2:28)

و هو الذى احياكم ثم يميتكم ثم يحييكم

It is He who gave you life then He makes you die,
then He brings you to life. (22:66)

There are a lot of other verses with the same meaning. In all of these instances, this ongoing observable system is mentioned as the system of creation. The opening of a seed under the ground, the growing of plants, and the bloom of trees in spring, are all mentioned as new and ongoing creations of God. Nowhere in the Qur'an do we see that the creation and God's will in creation have been limited to the first human being or animal that was created on earth. The Qur'an does not consider the first being as the only creation of God.

Although the story of Adam's creation has been mentioned first in the Holy Qur'an, this has not been to prove God's unity. Indeed, the Qur'an does not argue from the creation of Adam as the first human being for existence of God.

One of the Qur'an's wonders lies in the story of Adam. There the Qur'an elucidates a number of moral and educational teachings, including man's potential for being God's vicegerent on earth, man's potential in gaining knowledge, the humbleness of angels before this knowledge, man's ability to progress beyond the angels, the disadvantages of greed, the disadvantages of false pride, the role of committing sins in pulling man back from the high levels of perfection, the role of repentance in returning man to the position of God's vicinity, warning man against evil and seductive temptations, etc. However, the relation of Adam's miraculous creation to the issue of the unity of God and knowing the Creator has not been stated, since the reason behind telling the story has only been to give moral teachings rather than to view the beginning of life as evidence for proving the unity of God. Therefore, only the first human being is mentioned and the story of other animals and how their lives began is not mentioned.

We already noted that when monotheist scholars examine the first human, and want to justify how it gained life, they say that it has been created by God breathing His spirit into him. However, just as the life of the first human was created with being breathed into of God's spirit, the Holy Qur'an knows that the lives of other human beings which are born into this ongoing system have been created through the same process: the breath of spirit. At one point, regarding the issue of the first human, God says to the angels:

فاذا سويته و نفخت فيه من روحى فقعوا له ساجدين

So when I have proportioned him and breathed into him of My spirit, then fall down in prostration before him. (15:29)

At another point, He says:

و لقد خلقناكم ثم صورناكم ثم قلنا للملائكة اسجدوا لادم

Certainly We created you, then We formed you, then We said to the angels, 'Prostrate before Adam.' (7:11)

It is obvious in this verse that the creation, the breathing in of spirit and the prostration of angels is for all mankind. Elsewhere, He says:

الذى احسن كل شى ء خلقه و بدأ خلق الانسان من طين
ثم جعل نسله من سلالة من ماء مهين ثم سواه و نفخ فيه
من روحه و جعل لكم السمع و الابصار و الافئده لعلكم
تشكرون

who perfected everything that He created, and commenced man's creation from clay. Then He made his progeny from an extract of a base fluid. Then He proportioned them and breathed into him of His Spirit, and made for you the hearing, the sight, and the hearts. Little do you give thanks. (32:7-9)

As we understand from the verse above, and as the exegetes of the Qur'an have said, the pronoun in *"proportioned them"* refers to *"progeny"* and not to *"man."* [Of course, in English translation, this seems obvious since "them" cannot refer to "man," but in Arabic - which is the original language of the Qur'an - the pronoun used for both of them is the same. It is because of this point that the translator has interpreted the pronoun as progeny.]

It is important at this level to find out why - unlike the monotheist scholars who seek to discover the beginning of life when trying to relate life to God - the Qur'an does not consider any difference between the dawn of life and other periods of life, and realizes that life, even at its current level and progress, is the direct effect of God's will.

Indeed, the divergence between the Qur'an and the monotheist scholars is rooted in a more important difference. They seek God in the unknown periphery of their knowledge rather than from what can be known. Whenever they face something that is unknown, they look for God. They search for God in this unknown area of their knowledge. They always try to discover the secrets of issues for which they are not aware of their natural cause, and when they find themselves unable to find its cause, they relate it to God's will.

Therefore, the more natural causes are unknown to them, the more proofs they have for God's unity, and as their knowledge increases, their belief in God's unity decreases. For some believers, the supernatural is a storehouse for their unknown knowledge. Whatever is unknown to them, and for which they are not able to discover its natural cause, they relate to the supernatural. Wherever they think an exception has occurred, or the order of universe has been damaged, they consider it to be in the realm of the supernatural. Thus, whenever they cannot find the cause for a natural effect, they replace it with a supernatural cause, neglecting the fact that the supernatural itself has order and rules. Furthermore, when we replace a natural cause with another cause, the second one is also natural and at the same level of the first natural cause. The natural and the supernatural are in different levels and stand in a hierarchical order. Therefore, a natural cause cannot be replaced by a supernatural cause and vice versa.

Never in the Qur'an do we encounter a verse where an unknown cause has been mentioned as a proof of God's unity. Rather, the Qur'an mentions events in which man can recognise its natural cause and order and then takes the very same order as a proof.

Regarding life, the Qur'an views it as a grace beyond the realm of the sensible body which comes from a place higher than the physical world, whatever laws and procedures it may follow. Thus, the developments of life are developments of formation, coming into existence, creation and perfection. Of course, according to this logic, it makes no difference whether life has been created at once or gradually or one after another.

This logic is based on the fact that sensible matter has no life in its nature and that life is a grace and a light that has to be granted from a higher source. Therefore, the laws of life, in any form or shape, are the laws of creation.

The difference of the existential rank of matter and life is a scientific fact. In trying to discover the supernatural source of life, if we study this difference, we have used the positive side of our knowledge [i.e., what is known], rather than the negative [i.e., what is unknown]. We have sought God through our knowledge rather than through things which are unknown. Thus we will no longer need to degrade the supernatural by using it as an excuse whenever we are incapable of explaining a natural phenomenon. Rather, we can simply say that there must be a natural cause that we are not yet aware of.

Criticizing Fakhr al-Din Radi, Mulla Sadra in his *Al-Asfār al-Arba'ah* makes the same point by saying:

I wonder why when this man and people like him
want to prove the unity of God or another principle
of religion, they look in the realm of nature and try
to find something unknown, something that is out
of the universe's order.[2]

It can be understood from the above-mentioned verses of the
Qur'an that according to the Qur'anic perspective, creation does
not take place at once. An animal or a human, when moving in
the path of development, is constantly being created.
Furthermore, the whole universe is constantly being created and
is always in a state of incidence or flux. On the contrary, there is
another perspective that considers creation to have occurred in an
instant. Whenever theorists who hold this type of viewpoint want
to mention the creation of this universe, they look for that first
instant in which the universe was created from naught as if the
universe will not be a created creature if we do not consider it in
such a manner. Similarly, whenever these theorists want to prove
that life is created, they return to the first instant when life was
created. This is in line with what the Qur'an attributes to some
Jews who believed that God created the world in an instant and
then He retired. The Qur'an says:

و قالت اليهود يد الله مغلولة غلت ايديهم و لعنوا بما
قالوا...

The Jews say, 'God's hand is tied up.' Tied up be
their hands, and cursed be they for what they
say!... (5:64)

The standpoint about the relation between life and God's will that
always looks for the beginning of life in order to relate life to
God's will is rooted in the Jewish point of view mentioned above.
This idea spread over time throughout the world and has
unfortunately spread among some of the Muslim scholars as well.
However, we have said previously that, in the Qur'anic account,
there is no place for instant creation.

Before, we mentioned the challenges the world is facing today - Is man able to create a living organism? Is man able to create an artificial sperm that, when put inside a womb, can transform into a real person? We also mentioned that those who prove that life has been created by God, and held the beginning of life as a proof, deny this point and consider it to be impossible. However, according to the teachings that we receive from the Qur'an, it is not impossible. This issue needs more explanation and has to be considered from two different aspects.

One question we should consider is to notice how complicated the structure of a living organism is and if man will, one day, be able to discover the mysteries behind the combination of material parts and the formation of a living cell. We leave this to scientists to answer. They believe that what is more important and complicated than the creation of the earth, planets, galaxies and beings is the "protoplasm" (a semi-fluid, viscous, translucent colloid, the essential living matter of all animal and plant cells).

The second question we need to consider is, suppose one day man discovers the rule of the creation of living organism and finds all the conditions needed for it, and creates something exactly like a living organism. Will that artificial creature be given life? The answer is yes. Since it is impossible that all the conditions for granting life by God are ready and then life is not granted. Is it not that we believe God is the Absolute Perfect and the Absolute Granter? Is it not that the necessary-existent is necessary in all aspects, including granting life?

At this point, one might ask, have we not said that life is only due to God? Did we not believe that the giving and taking of life is beyond everyone's power except God? We mentioned earlier that the Qur'an has accepted this issue and the answer has become clear after the explanation we gave earlier about this issue. If man becomes capable of doing such, all he has done is to provide matter with the conditions of life, he has not created life. Man does not create life; rather it completes matter's ability for receiving life. Man is the mover, not the granter of existence.

Man, upon reaching that level, will have performed a great task in terms of science. However, even then his interference in the creation of life is as much as that of parents who give birth to a child, or a farmer who plants wheat. In none of these states does man create life. He provides matter with the conditions it needs for being granted life. This is how the Qur'an explains this fact and in the best way possible:

افرايتم ما تحرثون أ انتم تزرعونها ام نحن الزارعون

Have you considered what you sow? Is it you who makes it grow, or are We the grower? (56:63-63)

افرايتم ما تمنون أ انتم تخلقونه ام نحن الخالقون

Have you considered the sperm that you emit? Is it you who create it, or are We the creator? (56:58-59)

Now one might ask about the miracles of prophets. Indeed, they are beyond man's knowledge and power. The prophets have not achieved that level through ordinary means, rather they have been granted an extraordinary power and knowledge that took them above the normal levels of nature and which caused them to be able to perform such great feats.

If man achieves this level of scientific expertise, he has not yet done what the prophets did. They gave and took life by God's permission, however, all man can do is to prepare and provide the conditions needed for life to be given by God, just as man is able to provide the conditions for death but cannot take life. The giving and taking of life is only due to God, but man can prepare matter so that it is ready to be given life by God, or, on the other hand, remove this capability by discovering the rules for the giving and taking of life.

We have said that giving life is not an act of man and is beyond man's actions. Granting life and giving death are only done by God. We have also said that providing for life's conditions is man's role. Of course, it is not correct or even logical to conclude that man and God have divided duties, meaning some tasks are solely upon man to perform and God does not have any role in them and vice versa. Rather it is man's territory that is limited and dependant, not God's. Whatever is from God is absolute and infinite and whatever is limited and dependent is from man.[3]

---

[1] See e.g. Barroso, *History of Science*, p. 701.

[2] See *Usul-e Falsafeh wa Rawesh-e Realism*, vol. 3, p. 220.

[3] For further information in this regard, see *Usul-e Falsafeh wa Rawesh-e Realism*, vol. 5.

The Goodly Life from a Qur'anic Perspective

Hamid Mazaheri Seif

The Goodly Life (*al-Hayāt al-Tayyibah*) is a life which the Friends of Allah have obtained; they have earned its benefits as an outcome of moving towards God, serving Him and keeping the pledge that they have made to Him. It actualizes in the world-with-Him (the *'indallāh*-world) and with his mastership (*wilāyah*). The conditions of entering into that world are faith and patience in the struggle with the self (*nafs*) and its temptations. Its opposite is the delusional earthly life, which is based on polytheism (*shirk*), and confines the human being to a material life where Satan rules the self. This happens when the temptations control and enslave the *nafs*.

Introduction

Being the final and most perfect book sent by God for the guidance of mankind, the Holy Qur'an does not ignore anything regarding human progress and perfection. But since its audience is the whole of mankind and the majority of people are not very advanced in their level of guidance, the Qur'an indirectly points out the facts concerning the peaks of human perfection and eternal spiritual achievement. Accordingly, in order to discover its esoteric guidance, we need to examine the Qur'an closely in order to discover its deeper spiritual secrets.

One of the topics which has been indirectly pointed out in the Qur'an is the Goodly Life of the Friends of God. It has only been mentioned once, though explicitly, in verse 97 of *Surah al-Nahl*. However, there are further implicit mentions of the subject in other parts of the Qur'an, which draw a beautiful picture of the Goodly Life and the delicacies of its realization.

The Goodly Life of the Friends of Allah is a life without any kind of immorality. Through being in His presence and vicinity, it gives them the benefits of both this world and the Hereafter, benefits which are suitable to God's generosity.

This paper endeavours to explore the notion of the Goodly Life, and explains its different aspects in detail.

The Outline

The Qur'an says:

> Do not sell God's covenant for a paltry gain. Indeed, what is with God is better for you, should you know. That which is with you will be spent but what is with God shall last, and We will surely pay the patient their reward by the best of what they used to do. Whoever acts righteously, [whether] male or female, should he be faithful, we shall revive him with a Goodly Life and pay them their reward by the best of what they used to do. When you recite the Qur'an, seek the protection of God against the outcast Satan. Indeed, he does not have any authority over those who have faith and put their trust in their Lord. His authority is only over those who befriend him and those who make him a partner [of God]. (16:95-100)

There is a pledge between man and God, which, by its protection, opens the doors of spirituality to him. It joins man to Allah and the world-with-Him (the *'indallāh*-world); an eternal world in which life, happiness and achievement never cease. This recompense serves as a reward for the true believers, since they have not broken their pledge nor sold it cheaply; therefore, they are rewarded with greater than what they performed. This reward is called the Goodly Life; it is a life free of any deficiency, fear, failure, sadness or anything that can make life unpleasant. It is given to any man or woman as a result of acting righteously according to the faith. Hence, to achieve this bliss, we should seek the aid of divine revelation so that we can avoid the temptations of Satan, since he cannot have any influence on believers who trust in Allah. Opposed to this divine life is an inferior existence ruled by Satan and which is the fate of those who have committed polytheism (*shirk*) and accepted Satan's obedience.

One of the principal foundations of the aforementioned verses is the Goodly Life, of which different opinions are expressed. The late 'Allamah Tabarsi has stated some of these opinions on the meaning of the Goodly Life in *Majma' al-Bayān*, his prominent interpretation of the Qur'an, as follows:

- Having halal provisions

- An honourable life along with contentment and joy

- A happy life in the pleasant paradise

- A cheerful life in the *barzakhi* paradise[1]

In other interpretations of the Qur'an, "worshipping, along with having halal provision," "success upon obeying Allah," and similar terms are also mentioned as being part of the Goodly Life.[2]

While all these statements may be true, they only partially express the notion of the Goodly Life. None of them explains and analyses the Goodly Life using the verses which are mentioned before and after it. This study tries to expand on the meaning of the Goodly Life, by using the method of "interpretation of the Qur'an by Qur'an."

A Divine Covenant

In the aforementioned verses of *Surah al-Nahl*, keeping and fulfilling the Divine Covenant is presented as the key to entering the world-that-is-with-God (the *'indallah*-world) and earning its everlasting benefits:

> Do not sell God's covenant for a paltry gain. Indeed, what is with God is better for you, should you know. (3:95)

This covenant is the pledge that Allah took from every human after creating Adam and his descendants; He also made themselves the witnesses of this pledge:

> When your Lord took from the Children of Adam, from their loins, their descendants and made them bear witness over themselves, [He said to them,] 'Am I not your Lord?' They said, 'Yes indeed! We bear witness.' (7:172)

By bearing witness, the Qur'an means that man saw the reality of himself, which is the relation of his existence to God. And seeing this relation is knowing that his entire essence and existence is from God and depends on Him. In other words, when human beings saw themselves in the world-with-Allah, they found their existence to be completely from God, seeing themselves as slaves and perceiving His lordship.[3] We also find in Islamic traditions that every human being that has ever existed has known God when making his pledge.[4]

Ayatollah Javadi Amuli views this pledge as the *fitri* pledge of the human being to God and thus he recognizes the natural tendency of human beings towards God as the result of this pledge and the cognition of the reality of God.[5] However, the explanation of 'Allamah Tabataba'i seems more appropriate; the *fitrah*, being the unique inner instinct or intuition of human beings which was given to them by God, places the human in a special relationship with God and strengthens the tendency towards God-in-his-essence, which is in line with the spiritual aspect of human beings.

'Allamah Tabataba'i correlates this pledge with the heavenly aspect of human beings. He believes that heaven relates to the inner aspect of things which are directed towards God. Perceiving the pledge is associated with certitude (*yaqin*). In this regard, the Qur'an says:

> Thus did We show Abraham the dominions (*malakūt*) of the heavens and the earth, that he might be of those who possess certitude. (6:75)

What is meant by seeing the *"dominions of the heavens and the earth"* is not the material *thingness* of it, which results in the cognition of the properties of objects, rather it is their existential side which is dependent on, related to and in need of a God who controls everything. And He is the God of all creatures.[6] Before living in this inferior material world, man used to live in heaven and in the presence of God. There, he saw Him with all of His greatness, glory and beauty and testified to his lordship.

The testifying and acknowledgment of human beings to God's lordship leads to a pledge of not worshipping anything besides Him. The Qur'an expresses this fact in the following way:

> Did I not exhort you, O children of Adam, saying, 'Do not worship Satan. He is indeed your manifest enemy. Worship Me. That is a straight path?' (36:60; 36:61)

The other aspect of the unity of God's lordship is the unity of man's servitude to his master and lord. The Qur'an divides human beings into two groups in relation to the pledge:

1. People who abide by their pledge and worship and obey their lord.

> Only those who possess intellect take admonition.
> Those who fulfil God's covenant and do not break
> the pledge solemnly made, and those who join
> what God has commanded to be joined. (13:19-21)

2. People who break their pledge and defile themselves. They cause mischief on earth and obey Satan.

> But as for those who break God's compact after
> having pledged it solemnly, and sever what God
> has commanded to be joined, and cause corruption
> in the earth. It is such on whom the curse will lie,
> and for them will be the ills of the [ultimate]
> abode. (13:25)

The second group is further divided into two additional groups: those who still have an opportunity to correct themselves and those who have squandered all of their chances for reform. Finally, we have three types of people: honest people who maintain their pledge and act righteously, hypocrites who break their pledge yet still have time to repent and enter the circle of God's mercy, and lastly the hypocrites who are left with no chance of repentance. They will not be guided nor included within the mercy of God. These three groups have been described in the Qur'an as such:

> Among the faithful are men who fulfil what they
> have pledged to God. Of them are some who have
> fulfilled their pledge, and of them are some who
> still wait, and they have not changed in the least,
> that God may reward the true for their truthfulness,

and punish the hypocrites, if He wishes, or accept their repentance. Indeed, God is All-Forgiving, All-Merciful. (33:23-24)

Of course, the first rule for entering the world-with-Allah and achieving the Goodly Life is to retain one's loyalty to the pledge and not sell it for a cheap price.

The Little Value of the Worldly Life

Before mentioning that the Goodly Life is the reward of the pious, God says in the Qur'an:

> Do not sell God's covenant for a paltry gain. Indeed, what is with God is better for you, should you know. (16:95)

In this holy verse, two things are placed next to each other: "paltry gain" (*thamanan qalilan*) and "what is with God" (*mā 'indallah*). It is imperative to study both these phrases.

Upon further examining the Qur'an, it becomes obvious that "paltry gain" is in reality a description of this world. This idea of the low value of this world has also been presented as *"matā'"* (limited and mortal enjoyment or benefit) or, with even more emphasis, as *"matā'an qalilan"* (the very limited enjoyment or benefit[7]). Since this world, which is subject to alteration and destruction, is of little value, God says to his messenger:

> Say, 'The enjoyment of this world is little.' (4:77)

Sometimes the same notion has been mentioned in comparison with the eternality of the Hereafter:

> But the enjoyment of the life of this world compared with the Hereafter are but insignificant. (9:38)

The Qur'an warns us that it is through being satisfied with the little value of this life that man harms himself the most. However, our main problem is not the lack of knowledge about the mortality of this life. We sell our divine *fitrah* and our heavenly pledge, gaining the little value of this life, despite knowing the mortality of what we gain. So the question therefore is, why do we stick to this little value and forget the eternal and worthy blessings which are with God? In answering this question, the Qur'an describes the life of this world, which is in opposition to the Goodly Life:

> The life of this world is nothing but diversion and play. (29:64)

Play is an action or a group of activities that are performed unrealistically for an unrealistic purpose, similar to the playing of children.[8]

People envision the mortal pleasures of this world as something enormous and everlasting; therefore, they neglect God and the Hereafter. At this point, Satan makes these delusions stronger by utilising different methods to strengthen them in the heart of his followers and friends. Some of the methods that Satan uses are listed below:

Taswil: indicates taking something out of its genuine level and displaying it as much better than it actually is.[9] *"It was Satan who had seduced them."* (47:25)

Tazyin: presents something imperfect and defective as nice and decent. *"Satan had made to seem decorous to them what they had been doing."* (6:43)

Tamniah: means stimulating a desire for achieving a desired thing in the future, or in other words, stimulating one's wishes.[10] *"...[he] gives them [false] hopes, yet Satan does not promise them anything but delusion."* (4:120)

Ghurūr: neglects something because of something else.[11] *"Satan promises them nothing but delusion."* (17:64)

These techniques all make human beings refuse to see the incompleteness of this world. It is because of these deceptions, as well as his own whims, that he embraces the mortal pleasures of this world. The material life is, in fact, a delusional world that has been created for the non-believers and hypocrites by Satan. Therefore, the disapproved world which is the territory of Satan is not the natural world, but the delusional imaginary world that Satan's temptations create for everyone with the help of their own lower desires and appetites. On the other hand, the Goodly Life in the world-with-Allah actualizes for those who are honest.

The World-with-Allah:

From the verse 16:95 we can understand that keeping the pledge and promise to God brings forth a benefit from what-is-with-God. In other words, it is only through loyalty to the pledge that we can have the Goodly Life and be present in the world-with-Allah. The world-with-Allah - or according to great mystics, *"ālam-i 'indiyyat"*[12] - has some qualities which are also possessed by those who reach that heavenly world. The qualities of the world-with-Allah, and the qualities of those who enjoy the Goodly Life, are, in fact, the standards that indicate the difference between the benefits of the world-with-Allah and the trivial benefits of this world. The most important point about the world-with-Allah is that, like Allah himself, the world-with-Allah is not limited by time or place. One can experience and benefit from the Goodly Life by loyalty to the pledge. In this way, the glory and beauty of the world-with-Allah can be observed by man and he can live purely, in proximity to his Lord, having happiness, health, light, science, help, perfection and infinite blessings from God.

'Allamah Tabataba'i clarifies that the world-with-Allah does not precede this world in time; rather the world-with-Allah is dominant over this world and encompasses it.[13] Therefore, despite what some people may suppose, the world-with-Allah is not limited to the Hereafter. Indeed, its benefits include both this world and the Hereafter. These facts can be clearly understood through examining the Qur'an's verses.

The Characteristics of the Goodly Life and the World-with-Allah:

1. The Real Life

Those who enter the world-with-Allah earn the real life in the presence of Allah which is in fact the manifestation and effect of the divine name, "*al-Hayy*" (the living):

> They are living and provided for near their Lord. (3:169)

The fact that life in the world-with-Allah is genuine and that earthly life is delusional is not understood by the ignorant and the sinner until Judgment Day, when he says:

> 'Alas, had I sent ahead for my life!' (89:24)

Because it is the day when:

> ...the faithless are exposed to the Fire, [they will be told,] 'You have exhausted your good things in the life of the world and enjoyed them. So today you will be requited with a humiliating punishment for your acting arrogantly in the earth unduly, and because you used to transgress.' (46:20)

Perhaps the term "good things" (*tayyibāt*) in this verse refers to the heavenly pledge of serving Allah, which the unbelievers have violated in their earthy life and have therefore lost all its benefits and wasted all its opportunities. On Judgment Day, when they will face the true life and realize the vainness of their earthly life, they will cry out in regret.

2. The Gain of Both This Life and the Hereafter

The world-with-Allah is neither limited to the Hereafter nor to this life. Its gain includes both this world and the next and so the people who have gained entrance into the world-with-Allah benefit from its blessings and its rewards even in this world.[14]

> With God is the reward of this world and the Hereafter. (4:134)

In the supplications of the Imams, we also find another reference to this blessed life:

...و تحيينا حياة طيبة فى الدنيا والآخرة

> And revive us to a Goodly Life in both this life and the Hereafter![15]

It can here be understood that the Goodly Life includes the benefits of both this life and the Hereafter, and the above-mentioned verse says that the benefits of both lives are "with God." So the realization of the Goodly Life, which includes the gains of both lives, is in the world-with-Allah.

3. Permanency

The gain of the world-with-Allah is everlasting and can never decay or be destroyed. In the previously mentioned verses of *Surah al-Nahl*, after saying, *"Do not sell God's covenant for a paltry gain. Indeed, what is with God is better for you,"* the Holy Qur'an provides a reason for this: *"That which is with you will be spent but what is with God shall last."* We also see such similar phrases as:

> What is with God is better and more lasting. (28:60; 42:36)

101

4. The Unlimited World

The infinite source of everything is with God; and all the minute gains of this life are only beams radiating from that endless source.

> There is not a thing but that its sources are with Us, and We do not send it down except in a known measure. (15:21)

Therefore, the ones who enter the world-with-Allah have everything they desire without any restriction.

> They will have whatever they wish near their Lord. (39:34)[16]

> There they will have whatever they wish, and with Us there is yet more. (50:35)

5. The Existential Perfection

Entering the world-with-Allah is an essential change to perfection. People who achieve this are perfect by themselves and are the ranks of that world.

> They have ranks with God. (3:163)

That is, their perfection, qualities, gains and benefits do not come from an external factor apart from themselves; the movement towards reality has made them a source of perfection.

6. The Evaluation Scale

Since those who find their way to the world-with-Allah have climbed the peaks of perfection, that world and the people who have achieved its entrance, are the evaluation scale for the realities of this world.

> Indeed, the noblest of you in the sight of God is the most God-wary among you. (49:13)

...That is more just with God. (2:282; 33:5)

It can be understood from these verses that "the noblest" and "more just with God" are parts of the evaluation scale for things. Therefore the world-with-Allah and its realities are the evaluation scale for the realities of this world.

7. The Place for the Holy Books

The Holy Qur'an and other Divine Books are in the world-with-Allah and the people who enter that world see these sacred texts and understand their reality.

> And when there came to them a Book from God. (2:89)

> Indeed, you receive the Qur'an from One who is All-Wise, All-Knowing. (27:6)

Other than the Holy Qur'an, other Holy Books - or at least some levels of the Divine Book - are in the world-with-Allah.

> And with Him is the Mother of the Book. (13:39)

> And with Us is a preserving Book. (50:4)

> And indeed, it is with Us in the Mother Book [and it is] surely sublime and wise. (43:4)

These books contain all the realities of the world, from the life stories of the righteous and the bad people to all the events of the world. They are safe with Allah and those who are close to Him and the people of the world-with-Allah see them.

> The record of the pious is indeed in 'Illiyūn. And what will show you what is 'Illiyūn? It is a written record, witnessed by those brought near [to God]. (83:18-21)

8. The Display of the Divine Signs

The world-with-Allāh contains the explicit display of His signs.

> The signs are only with God. (6:109; 29:50)

Only those who have journeyed to the world-with-Allāh can understand His signs. Everything in this world is a sign of God for those who have seen Him and have realized His connection with the phenomena of the world. We usually assume that it is through these signs that we should understand God and that these signs are a reason for the cognition of God, yet this cognition is not precise or adequate because, in fact, He is the reason for the phenomena of the world, and only by knowing Him and understanding His presence can we can have a true knowledge of His signs. Those who are revived to the Goodly Life and who have achieved the world-with-Allāh, first perceive God and then, only later, become aware of His display in His signs.[17] Consequently, they recognize all of His signs to be in existence with Him, and hence understand the true meaning of "sign." Thus we have the following in the Holy Qur'an:

> Soon We shall show them Our signs in the horizons and in their own souls until it becomes clear to them that He is the Real. Is it not sufficient that your Lord is witness to all things? Look! They are indeed in doubt about the encounter with their Lord! Look! He indeed comprehends all things! (41:53-54)

In *Risālah al-Wilāyah*, 'Allamah Tabataba'i maintaines that the pronoun in the phrase *"annahu'l-haqq"* refers to God. Tabataba'i also considers the word *"shahid"* (witness) to mean *"mashhūd"* (being witnessed). Therefore, according to Tabataba'i, this verse indicates that that everything which a human being initially sees is first God and then the thing which He created because He who is obvious does not leave a place for the obscure.[18] In fact, His signs are a reminder to us of our pre-existent *fitri* pledge to someone we have seen and known. Thus, His signs do not necessarily have to be proven to anyone with logical reasoning except to those who have made their minds impure and blocked with doubts. His signs are simply reminders that represent His displays.[19]

9. Knowledge

"Knowledge," in the Qur'an, is the cognition of Allah and His signs.[20] Indeed, the Holy Qur'an states that all knowledge is with God.

> Knowledge is with God alone. (46:23)

Therefore, anyone who attains the real knowledge gains benefit from Allah and finds a way to the world-with-Allah.

> ...And [We] taught him a knowledge from Our own Presence. (18:65)

Therefore, knowledge is one of the greatest characteristics of the Goodly Life and of the people who have achieved this life. The Household of the Prophet Muhammad (s) are the source of this knowledge and the pioneers of the people who have attained the Goodly Life. Imam Baqir (a) has said:

> I swear to God, we are God's treasurers on earth; not the treasurers of gold and silver, but the treasurers of His knowledge.[21]

10. Light

Only those who have purified their souls and forsaken all their worldly attachments, interests and dependencies can find a way to the Goodly Life. Allah accepts these people to be with Him and gives them success in realizing the world-with-Allah.

> Those who have faith in God and His apostles, it is they who are the truthful and the witnesses with

their Lord; they shall have their reward and their light. (57:19)

These are the people who have understood Allah with all their capacity and have acted as a mirror for His light. They live among the people with this light and are a source of guidance for them.

> Is he who was lifeless, then We gave him life and provided him with a light by which he walks among the people, like the one who dwells in a manifold darkness which he cannot leave? (6:122)

Anyone who has advanced to the world-with-Allah reflects the light of Allah according to his capacity, but the Household of the Prophet (s) perceive and reflect His light and brighten the world in a complete manner. Abu Khālid Kabuli reports that he asked Imam Baqir (a) about the verse, *"So have faith in God and His Apostle and the light which We have sent down..."* (64:8). Imam answered:

> O Abu Khālid, I swear to God, "light" is the Imams from the generation of the Prophet until Judgment Day. And I swear to God, they are the light of God that is sent down. And I swear to God, the light of the Imams in the heart of faithful is more than the light of the sun. And I swear to God, they have brightened the souls of the faithful and Allah the Almighty hides their light from whoever He desires so that his soul is darkened.[22]

11. The Place of the Truth

Those who neglect the signs sent by God will fall into Satan's trap and be ensnared by the false delusions created by him:

Whoever turns a blind eye to the remembrance of the All-Beneficent, We assign him a devil who remains his companion. (43:36)

In contrast to this is the secure, unwavering and rightful position of people who have attained the Goodly Life. They live *"in the abode of truthfulness with an Omnipotent King"* (54:55) and, because their belief leaves no place for delusion, there is no room for Satan. God says to his Prophet: *"Give good news to the faithful that they are in the abode of truthfulness with their Lord"* (10:2), which means that they will find the true path, obtain the true position and live with rightness, rather than with deceptions and mirages.

12. Servitude

Servitude means the possession of one intelligent creature by another. God, who is the owner of everything, is served by all humans, angels, and other intelligent creatures. One who does not accept servitude of this kind is indeed arrogant. Only people who consider their life to be a possession of God, and clear their mind and thoughts from arrogance, can find a way to the world-with-Allah. The Qur'an says:

And those who are near Him do not disdain to worship Him, nor do they become weary. (21:19)

Without a doubt, it is the abidance by and loyalty to the pledge that elevates the believers to a level where they experience the Goodly Life and obtain the true position. On the other hand, the delusions and deceptions of the followers of Satan all begin with untruthfulness and the breaking of the *fitri* pledge.

13. Extraordinary Power

When Zechariah went to the sanctuary to visit Mary and saw the fresh fruits that were there, he asked: *"O Mary, from where does this come to you?"* To which she replied, *"It comes from God."* (3:37) People who have gained the Goodly Life benefit from infinite treasures and are supported by the power and wealth of God, for they have reached the highest levels of the world-with-Him. Therefore, they can perform extraordinary acts (*karāmat*) that normal people are unable to perform.

14. Special Provision

Those who have attained the Goodly Life experience blessings in the world-with-Allah that are beyond our imagination.

> They are living and provided for near their Lord.
> (3:169)

This provision not only consists of nourishment, clothing and beautiful gardens but also special blessings that enliven hearts and make the Goodly Life continue in the world-with-Allah.

15. Help

The most difficult challenge that man confronts arises when Satan's temptations, as well as his own lower desires and appetites, conspire together to compel him to neglect God and preoccupy him with this material world. In these times, only God can help man.

> And victory comes only from God. (3:126)

When brothers and friends are not able to be of any assistance, it is only God who can help man not to be caught up in the materialistic life and make mistakes that prevent him from perceiving the presence of God. Therefore, those who have attained the Goodly Life are protected from committing sins, and because of their decent life, which is a direct result of their combat with the lower self (*nafs*), God's mercy and grace embrace them. And even if they commit a sin unintentionally, they will repent immediately and become released from its evilness.

16. Special Mercy

God's general mercy includes everything and everyone, encompassing both believers and nonbelievers. However, His special mercy, which is only for the world-with-Allah, includes people who live the Goodly Life. God says in the Qur'an about Prophet Khiḍr that *"We had granted him a mercy from Ourselves"* (18:65) or, in another verse about Prophet Job (*Ayyūb*) after the difficult test he passed, when divine blessings were given back to him: *"And We gave him [back] his family along with others like them, as a mercy from Us"* (21:84). In another verse, God quotes Noah: *"He has granted me His own mercy."* (11:28)

God's special mercy actualizes in different ways; the knowledge of Khiḍr, the return of Job's health and wealth in an amazing way and the Prophethood of Noah are all examples of God's special mercy that have been granted to them since they have been perfectly guided.

Therefore, special mercy is granted when the divine guidance has proven effective and man reaches the valuable position of servitude. This is the point when he reaches the world-with-Allah and attains the Goodly Life. The Lord's general mercy is both a means and an opportunity for guidance, yet if it is used inappropriately, it will result in God's anger and if used properly, its outcome will be His special mercy.

17. Reward of the Righteousness

Although, in the Hereafter, the world-with-Allah will be unveiled and the righteous receive their complete reward after their death when they pass from this world, they are actually joyful in both worlds. Because of being in the world-with-Allah and having achieved the Goodly Life, they feel happy, safe and tranquil because of their close relation with God. The Qur'an says:

They shall have their reward near their Lord, and they will have no fear, nor will they grieve. (2:162)

There are many other verses that refer to the same fact.[23]

18. Punishment of the Sinful

The world-with-Allah is the Hereafter and the resurrection and it is through passing by the earthly pleasures and by being equipped with the power of certitude that those who live the Goodly Life can perceive it right now. The Qur'an says:

No indeed! Were you to know with certain knowledge, you would surely see hell. (102:5-6)

The sinful who are negligent, and therefore may enjoy themselves in this world, will be punished because of their false beliefs and bad deeds as soon as they are present before God on Judgement Day.

Soon the guilty will be visited by a degradation before God and a severe punishment because of the plots they used to devise. (6:124)

...when the guilty hang their heads before their Lord... (32:12)

19. The Hereafter

Considering the last two qualities, we can conclude that the world-with-Allah is none other than the Hereafter (*ākhirah*). Of course, other qualities like permanency also point this out. The Qur'an says: *"while the Hereafter is better and more lasting."* (87:17)

Furthermore, the Qur'an itself clearly mentions that the Hereafter is with God: *"If the abode of the Hereafter with God were exclusively for you, and not for other people, then long for death, should you be truthful"* (2:94) and *"...and the Hereafter near your Lord is for the Godwary"* (43:35). The Hereafter therefore is the world-with-Allah, and those who are revived to the Goodly Life live as if they observe Judgement Day and its collective rewards and punishments even if they still have a material presence in the natural world.[24]

The Hereafter is present now; however, the veil of earthly delusions prevents us from seeing the internal aspect (*bātin*) of this world which is Hereafter. The Qur'an says:

> They know just an outward aspect of the life of
> the world, but they are oblivious of the Hereafter.
> (30:7)

Thus, the Hereafter exists hidden beyond the earth and sky[25] and when Judgement Day arrives the veils will be removed from everyone's eyesight so that they will be able to see:

> You were certainly oblivious of this. We have
> removed your veil from you, and so your sight is
> acute today. (50:22)

20. Salām

"Salām" means being healthy and free from any kind of disease or deficiency. Those who have achieved the Goodly Life and are in the world-with-Allah are symbols representing one of God's names, *Salām*. They are immune and protected from all illnesses. The Qur'an says:

> For them shall be the abode of peace near their
> Lord and He will be their guardian. (6:127)

This immunity is not only in regards to one's body; it is also the immunity of the spirit and heart since in the eternal life it is the spirit that is significant, not the body. Thus we read in the Qur'an:

The day when neither wealth nor children will avail, except him who comes to God with a sound heart. (26:88-89)

On the contrary, for those who have not achieved the world-with-Allah and who do not possess the Goodly Life, Allah says:

There is a sickness in their hearts; then God increased their sickness, and there is a painful punishment for them. (2:10)

These sick hearts will not even understand the presence of God on Judgment Day as He deserves and this might be their worst punishment on that day.

But whoever disregards My remembrance, his shall be a wretched life, and on the Day of Resurrection We shall raise him blind. He will say, 'My Lord! Why have You raised me blind, though I used to see?' He will say: 'So it is. Our signs came to you, but you forgot them, and thus you will be forgotten today.' (20:124-126)

Patience Prepares One for Entering the World-with-Allah and Achieving the Goodly Life

Regarding the reward of the patient, the Qur'an says:

مَا عِندَكُمْ يَنفَدُ وَمَا عِندَ اللَّهِ بَاقٍ وَلَنَجْزِيَنَّ الَّذِينَ صَبَرُوا أَجْرَهُم بِأَحْسَنِ مَا كَانُوا يَعْمَلُونَ

That which is with you will be spent but what is with God shall last, and We will surely pay the patient their reward by the best of what they used to do. (16:96)

The reward of the righteous who reach the world-with-Allah is much greater than their levels of patience - to the extent that it

112

might not be counted as the reward for their patience. However, their patience has been the basis for entering the world-with-Allah and having the Goodly Life and consequently benefiting from its great rewards.

Indeed, this holy verse has deemed patience as the basis for entering the world-with-Allah and has not mentioned any other virtues. This is because patience and forbearance are the basis for a firm determination in struggling against the lower self. Patience finds its meaning when the lower self confronts the *fitrah*, the inclination to the earthly life struggles with that of the world-with-Allah, and then by patience and the keeping of the divine pledge, the lower self is defeated, leaving the inclination to the world-with-Allah victorious. This is why in the hadith of *Mi'rāj* the state of people who have the *ākhirah* is described thus:

يموت الناس مرّة و يموت احدهم فى كل يوم سبعين مرّة من مجاهدة انفسهم و مخالفة هواهم و الشيطان الذى يجرى فى عروقهم ... فوّعزتى و جلالى لاحيينّهم حياة طيّبة

People die one time, but those who remember *ākhirah*, each die seventy times each day in struggle with their nafs and conflict with their desires and the Satan that is in their vessels. By my honour and glory, I will revive them to the Goodly Life.[26]

In order to achieve the Goodly Life and exist in the world-with-Allah, one has to remove his inner dependencies and interests of this world, and this can only be done by being patient regarding the servitude pledge. This will release the heart from the cage of this world, and then, before natural death, those who are patient will have the Goodly Life. Imam Ali (a) said:

اخرجوا من الدنيا قلوبكم قبل ان تخرّج منها ابدانكم

113

Take your hearts out of this world before your
bodies are taken out.[27]

Prophet Muhammad said:

موتوا قبل ان تموتوا

Die before you die.[28]

Or another statement from him :

بموت النفس يكون حياة القلب

The heart is revived through the death of the lower self
(*nafs*).[29]

This death, or spiritual martyrdom, is the basis for a better and
more purified life. They free their lives from darkness and
separate their hearts and spirits from the life of this world. They
have reached the world of light, help, mercy, health, infinity and
eternality which is the world-with-Allah. And God manifests His
attributes in them. Indeed, all of these great rewards are the
results of struggling and having power over the *nafs*. This is why
God said in the Qur'an:

وَلَنَجْزِيَنَّ الَّذِينَ صَبَرُوا أَجْرَهُم بِأَحْسَنِ مَا كَانُوا يَعْمَلُونَ

We will surely give those who were patient their reward
according to the best of what they used to do. (16:96)

Zayd ibn Arqam narrates from Imam Husayn (a) that he said:

ما من شيعتنا الا صدّيق شهيد. قلت: انّى يكون ذلك و
هم يموتون على فراشهم؟ فقال: اما تتلوا كتاب الله
((والذين ءامنوا بالله و رسله اولئك هم الصديقون و
الشهداء عند ربهم)) ثم قال: لو لم تكن الشهادة الّا لمن
قتل بالسيف لاقلّ الله الشهداء

114

There is no follower of us except that he is truthful and martyr (or witness). Zayd then said: "How is that possible while they may die in their bed (i.e. naturally)?" Imam replied: "Haven't you recited God's book which says: *'Those who have faith in God and His apostles - it is they who are the truthful and the martyrs* (or witnesses) *with their Lord...'*[30] And if martyrdom was only for those who got killed by swords, the martyrs would be really few."[31]

In this narration, and also in the holy verse mentioned above, the world-with-Allah and the state of being in that world have been mentioned and the spiritual martyrdom of the believers who have reached the high levels of faith and are present in the world-with-Allah have been emphasised. Here it might be appropriate to mention a few verses of a poem composed by Ibn Fāriḍ:

> *If you want a calm life, live without passion. For the lovers' relief is pain and hardship. It starts with soreness and ends with getting killed.*

> *But if you want a blissful life, sacrifice yourself in Love and then you're a martyr. Otherwise leave it, since the burning passion of the enthusiastic has its own devotees. As one has to endure the bite of a bee to get to the sweet honey, those who don't die in love don't grow and progress. Say to the martyrs of love, "You did well in expressing your love." And say to the claimants, "A kohl painted eye is never like a black eye."*[32]

The ordinary people know two kinds of *jihād*; one being the minor struggle (*al-jihād al-asghar*), fighting with an external enemy, and the other, greater struggle (*al-jihād al-akbar*), fighting the internal temptations to commit sins. But the superior people and the people of the Goodly Life know three kinds of *jihāds*. Fighting against their temptations in order to not commit sin is their middle *jihād*. Their greatest struggle and combat is

115

with their own *nafs* and the illusion of considering themselves apart from Allah. When someone wins this fight, he dies for Allah and then is revived to the Goodly Life at its most perfect level.

Faith Is the Condition for the Goodly Life

Faith is a requirement for achieving the Goodly Life. That is, by having faith, the Goodly Life can be achieved and anyone who has enough faith most definitely has attained the Goodly Life. By having more faith, higher levels of the Goodly Life can then be reached. God says in the Qur'an:

مَنْ عَمِلَ صَالِحًا مِّن ذَكَرٍ أَوْ أُنثَىٰ وَهُوَ مُؤْمِنٌ فَلَنُحْيِيَنَّهُ حَيَاةً طَيِّبَةً وَلَنَجْزِيَنَّهُمْ أَجْرَهُم بِأَحْسَنِ مَا كَانُوا يَعْمَلُونَ

Whoever acts righteously, [whether] male or female, should he be faithful, We shall revive him with a good life and pay them their reward by the best of what they used to do. (16:97)

From this verse and the verse preceding it, it can be concluded that the benefit of the world-with-Allah that is given to those who have faith and act righteously is the Goodly Life. Because in verse 96, the eternality of the world-with-Allah is mentioned prior to the reward of the patient and their reward is described as "the best of what they used to do." In verse 97, the meaning of patience is demonstrated; faith is its foundation which leads to righteous deeds. At the end of the verse, the reward is mentioned once again. Therefore, verse 97 is the explanation of verse 96, and also its emphasis; thus these two verses are associated with each other. Indeed, we have the explanation of "الَّذِينَ صَبَرُوا" (*Those who are patient*), in the next verse with "مِّن ذَكَرٍ أَوْ أُنثَىٰ" (*male or female*) and "مَا عِندَ اللَّهِ بَاقٍ" (*What is with God shall last*) is also clarified with "فَلَنُحْيِيَنَّهُ حَيَاةً طَيِّبَةً" (*We shall revive him with a Good Life*). Additionally, the pronouns referring to Allah change in these two verses from the third person singular to the first person plural in the Arabic version, which shows the regard and importance of the Goodly Life.

In this holy verse, righteous deeds - an obvious instance of which would be patience in serving Allah and struggle with *nafs* – are considered as the initiator of the Goodly Life and its condition is considered to be faith. The cognition of God and the tendency towards Him are the two columns of faith[33] which guide the understanding and will of human beings towards Allah. These two aspects of humanity, which surround his essence, lead him towards joining the pure world of God's lordship. It is then, in His Holy Presence, that human beings find another life. It is like he is born again to a world, to which the material world by comparison is just like the mother's womb to the material world. Jesus Christ (a) has said:

لن يلج ملكوت من لم يولد مرتين

> One who has not been born twice does not find a way to the kingdom of God (*malakūt*).[34]

When the heart of a believer is released from the limitations of this world, and he flies to the sky of God's Holy Lordship with the wings of "faith" and "virtue," letting go of this world, His heart and his soul are expanded into a vast world that contains the Godly Heavens. Our Holy Prophet (s) has said:

قلب المومن عرش الرحمن

> The heart of a believer is the heaven of the beneficent God.[35]

Of course, this type of faith is very high in level which can make the heart of a believer the place of God's manifestation. Like light, faith has different levels of brightness. The faith of some people is so slight that it cannot completely brighten their hearts from darkness. But there are people whose faith shines like the

117

sun: the dignity of their faith and the light of their life brightens cold and dark hearts.

Levels of Faith

Scholars have ascertained four levels of faith:[36]

1. Having general belief in the meaning of "*shahādatayn*" (when a person witnesses to God's lordship and Prophet Muhammad's prophethood) which requires performing the majority of the practices of Islam. Committing some types of sins does not conflict with this level of faith.

2. Having detailed belief in religious facts. God says about this group of believers that:

إِنَّمَا الْمُؤْمِنُونَ الَّذِينَ آمَنُوا بِاللَّهِ وَرَسُولِهِ ثُمَّ لَمْ يَرْتَابُوا وَجَاهَدُوا بِأَمْوَالِهِمْ وَأَنْفُسِهِمْ فِي سَبِيلِ اللَّهِ أُولَٰئِكَ هُمُ الصَّادِقُونَ '

> The faithful are only those who have attained faith in God and His Apostle and then have never doubted, and who wage jihad with their possessions and their persons in the way of God. It is they who are the truthful. (49:15)

3. This level of faith is achieved only by complete submission to the will of God and His Messenger. The beginning verses of *Surah al-Muminūn* is about this issue and all the accomplished moralities are the fruit and gain of this level of faith. In fact, at this level of faith, the believer sees the whole world as the possession of God and does not find himself beyond God's power and dominion. Thus, he submits himself completely to God and tries to earn everything which is good since he sees himself as a possession of God and acts according to what He wants.

4. It is at this level of faith that the believer truly understands the reality of God's ownership and realizes that this does not

resemble the ownership of man. Nothing is independent before God and everything, including its essence, qualities and actions, is dependent on Him and is in absolute reverence to Him. At this level, the faithful grasps unity of God in His essence and in ownership, delusions are eliminated and he sees nothing but the face of Allah and understands the meaning of the verse:

$$\text{كُلُّ شَيْءٍ هَالِكٌ إِلَّا وَجْهَهُ}$$

Everything perishes except His Face. (28:88)

When the heart is in this state, the believer becomes one of God's friends, about whom He has said:

$$\text{أَلَا إِنَّ أَوْلِيَاءَ اللَّهِ لَا خَوْفٌ عَلَيْهِمْ وَلَا هُمْ يَحْزَنُونَ الَّذِينَ}$$
$$\text{آمَنُوا وَكَانُوا يَتَّقُونَ}$$

Look! The friends of God will indeed have no fear nor will they grieve, for those who have faith, and are Godwary. (10:62-63)

The Goodly Life and the Mastership of God

The Goodly Life actualizes in the world-with-Allah under His mastership by means of the condition of faith. The Qur'an says:

$$\text{اللَّهُ وَلِيُّ الَّذِينَ آمَنُوا يُخْرِجُهُم مِّنَ الظُّلُمَاتِ إِلَى النُّورِ}$$

God is the Master of the Faithful: He brings them out of darkness into light. (2:257)

The term "darkness" in this verse might refer to the delusions of this world whereas the term "light" may refer to the world-with-Allah and, as with previous explanations, the reason for this conclusion is clear. In another verse, God says:

$$\text{وَاللَّهُ وَلِيُّ الْمُؤْمِنِينَ}$$

God is the guardian of the faithful. (3:68)

Without any doubt, as the level of faith rises, so does the level of the mastership of God, and at the peaks of faith and mastership, one becomes able to understand the presence of the world-with-Allah.

The mastership of God reaches mankind both directly from God and through His Greatest Friends, whose mastership is God's mastership.

إِنَّمَا وَلِيُّكُمُ اللَّهُ وَرَسُولُهُ وَالَّذِينَ آمَنُوا الَّذِينَ يُقِيمُونَ الصَّلَاةَ وَيُؤْتُونَ الزَّكَاةَ وَهُمْ رَاكِعُونَ

Your guardian is only God, His Apostle, and the faithful who maintain the prayer and give the alms while bowing down. (5:55)

There is an important point in this verse and that is the singularity of the term "guardian" which indicates that the mastership of the Prophet and the Faithful is the same as God's mastership. Thus we understand that the masterships of the Faithful and the Prophet are only manifestations of God's mastership and not anything independent from it.

According to the authentic hadiths, the faithful who have been mentioned in this verse after the Prophet are Imam Ali[37] and his eleven Infallible Successors. Their mastership over believers is a manifestation of God's mastership. Thus they have certain rights over the believers. Abu Basir says:

انّ المؤمنَ اذا ماتَ رأى رسول الله و عليّاً يحضُرانه و قال رسول الله: أَنَا أَحد الوالدين و عليٌّ الآخرقالَ: قلت: و أيُّ موضع ذلك من كتابِ الله؟ قالَ: قوله "اعبدوالله و لا تُشرَكوا به شيئاً و بالوالدين احساناً"

I heard Imam Sadiq (a) saying: "Truly, when a believer dies he sees Prophet Muhammad and Imam Ali (a) present there. The Apostle of God said: 'I am one parent and Ali (a) is the other one.'" Then Abu Basir asked Imam Sadiq: "Where in the Qur'an has this been said?" Imam replied: "Where Allah says, 'Worship God and do not ascribe any partners to Him, and be good to your parents' (4:36).[38]

'Allamah Majlesi explains this narration saying, "Man has a physical life with an animal spirit and an eternal life with faith, knowledge and spiritual perfections which results in never-ending happiness. Definitely, in different verses of the Qur'an, God has referred to the polytheists as dead. On the other hand, He has described believers who have died as alive. As He has said:

$$\text{وَلَا تَحْسَبَنَّ الَّذِينَ قُتِلُوا فِي سَبِيلِ اللَّهِ أَمْوَاتًا ۚ بَلْ أَحْيَاءٌ عِندَ رَبِّهِمْ يُرْزَقُونَ}$$

Do not suppose those who were slain in the way of God to be dead; rather they are living and provided for near their Lord. (3:169)

Similar concepts can be found throughout the Qur'an and the Prophetic traditions.

Fulfilling the rights of blood parents is obligatory because we owe them with respect to our earthly lives, but the right of Prophets and Imams are obligatory from two perspectives:

First, they are the reason for which God created everything, and all the creatures are protected and provided for because of them. Hence, they are the reason for the existence of the universe.

And second, due to their guidance towards a greater life that people benefit from and thus earn the Goodly Life under their light."

Therefore, they are our spiritual fathers and fulfilling their rights is an obligatory task.[39] The Goodly Life is under the mastership of Allah which actualizes through the mastership of the Prophet and His Household.

The Outcomes of the Goodly Life:

The outcomes of the Goodly Life are countless. Those who earn it gain a great happiness for being with Allah, in His proximity, and their hearts manifest and reflect Godly qualities.

The greatest gain of the Goodly Life is the encountering of Allah in the world-with-Allah, which is reserved for His friends.

$$\text{فَمَن كَانَ يَرْجُو لِقَاءَ رَبِّهِ فَلْيَعْمَلْ عَمَلًا صَالِحًا وَلَا يُشْرِكْ بِعِبَادَةِ رَبِّهِ أَحَدًا}$$

> So whoever expects to encounter his Lord, let him act righteously, and not associate anyone with the worship of his Lord. (18:110)

In this verse, the encountering of Allah is introduced under the two principles of "acting righteously" and "not committing polytheism," or simply being faithful. Hence, earning the Goodly Life comes under these conditions as well.

Therefore, both the Goodly Life and the encountering of Allah are the results of faith and righteous deeds, and because life is the source of motion and sensation in living beings, those who earn the Goodly Life and have developed their souls gain a deep level of understanding that can encounter God and see His light. Their hearts are not dead like stones and so they readily grasp the lights of God. The Qur'an says:

$$\text{فَإِنَّكَ لَا تُسْمِعُ الْمَوْتَىٰ}$$

> Indeed, you cannot make the dead hear. (30:52)

$$\text{لِّيُنذِرَ مَن كَانَ حَيًّا}$$

So that anyone who is alive may be warned.
(36:70)

Thus, encountering of God in lower levels leads to progress on the path, thus giving life to the true believers, and finally leading to a more perfect encountering of God.

The friends of Allah understand the interior world and the Goodly Life and perceive it's mysteries with purified hearts.

$$\text{إِنَّ فِي ذَٰلِكَ لَذِكْرَىٰ لِمَن كَانَ لَهُ قَلْبٌ أَوْ أَلْقَى السَّمْعَ وَهُوَ شَهِيدٌ}$$

There is indeed an admonition in that for one who
has a heart, or gives ear, being attentive. (50:37)

Although their actions resemble the actions of others, they have strong understanding, sense and determination that originate from another source, which is the pure human life. These people, aside from having the qualities of animal life, have another life that the unbelievers do not have - the human life.

One of the other results of the Goodly Life is inner happiness and peace. In describing the friends of Allah and the people who have obtained the Goodly Life, the Qur'an says:

$$\text{أَلَا إِنَّ أَوْلِيَاءَ اللَّهِ لَا خَوْفٌ عَلَيْهِمْ وَلَا هُمْ يَحْزَنُونَ الَّذِينَ آمَنُوا وَكَانُوا يَتَّقُونَ}$$

Look! The friends of God will indeed have no fear
nor will they grieve. Those who have faith, and are
Godwary. (10:62-63)

In another verse, it says:

إِنَّ الَّذِينَ آمَنُوا وَالَّذِينَ هَادُوا وَالصَّابِئُونَ وَالنَّصَارَىٰ مَنْ
آمَنَ بِاللَّهِ وَالْيَوْمِ الْآخِرِ وَعَمِلَ صَالِحًا فَلَا خَوْفٌ عَلَيْهِمْ وَلَا
هُمْ يَحْزَنُونَ

> Indeed the faithful, the Jews, the Sabaeans, and the
> Christians those who have faith in God and the
> Last Day and act righteously they will have no
> fear, nor will they grieve. (5:69)

Man fears the things he might face that could spoil his happiness
and he grieves when something transpires which does ruin his
happiness. Yet fear never occurs if man and what belongs to him
are immune from any danger, and similarly he will never grieve if
he is blessed and has an absolutely happy life which will not be
subject to any harm. This is the eternality of happiness for man
and the eternality of man in happiness.

When man's heart is free of all affinities except for the propensity
towards God and his heart is filled with light and the awareness
of God, he is then allowed near God and to the world-with-Allah
and thus he will be prosperous and have obtained the better and
eternal life. 'Allamah Tabataba'i says:

> God, in his Holy Book, has said that the divine
> men have an eternal life which doesn't end with
> their death, and it is secure even after their death
> under the mastership of God. There is no place for
> difficulty and exhaustion in that life nor is there
> place for abjection and misery. People who live
> that life are surrounded by God's love and are
> pleased to be near Him. They face nothing but
> happiness. They have safety, health, exhilaration,
> and pleasures which are not mixed with any kind
> of fear, danger or destruction. They see and hear
> things which others are incapable of seeing and
> hearing and their wisdom and their will are far
> above that of the others.[40]

Therefore, from the results which can be obtained in the Goodly Life, what is more important than happiness and peace is the superior sense and insight which reveals what is beyond this world and the *malakūt* (dominion; kingdom) of the skies and the earth for the dignified believers. This ability and insight is a manifestation of God's light which has glowed into their hearts and has made them deep and wide. As a result they have come out of the darkness of seeing only appearances and have entered the light of seeing the interior aspect of things and thus have found another life.

يَا أَيُّهَا الَّذِينَ آمَنُوا اتَّقُوا اللَّهَ وَآمِنُوا بِرَسُولِهِ يُؤْتِكُمْ كِفْلَيْنِ مِن رَّحْمَتِهِ وَيَجْعَل لَّكُمْ نُورًا تَمْشُونَ بِهِ

"O you who have faith! Be wary of God and have faith in His Apostle. He will grant you a double share of His mercy and give you a light to walk by. (57:28)

There are numerous mysteries hidden in this verse. It tells the believers to have faith, and by faith, the high levels of faith are meant; otherwise the verse does not make sense. The believers already have a certain level of faith and telling them to have faith again is the same as ordering them to acquire something which has already been acquired, which is not only impossible but also useless. And we know that God does not order vainly. However, the qualification for obtaining these high levels and the way of achieving them is through God-consciousness and righteous acts. Further in the verse, He says if you are faithful and wary of God you will be granted two blessings. Out of these two blessings, which come from God's mercy, one might be the primary encountering of Allah which is the result of faith, and the other might be martyrdom, which is the result of God-consciousness and struggling with the *nafs*. And these two are the basis of the light that Allah grants the believers and which is called the Goodly Life. When He mentioned *"a light to walk by,"* He used walking as a symbol of life and all its activities; which means that the normal life and all of the activities of those who live the Goodly Life have a special profoundness even though they are living a normal life. They benefit from a conferred light and a special life; they walk and do everything by that light. They see God before seeing anything and have no intention except to please Him.

Seeking the Protection of God

The Qur'an says:

فَإِذَا قَرَأْتَ الْقُرْآنَ فَاسْتَعِذْ بِاللَّهِ مِنَ الشَّيْطَانِ الرَّجِيمِ

> When you recite the Qur'an, seek the protection of God against the outcast Satan. (16:98)

The Qur'an is the best outcome of Prophet Muhammad's journey towards God and the best gift given by God to His Friends. It is through this revelation that God keeps the righteous people in His mastership. Thus, He orders His Prophet to say:

إِنَّ وَلِيِّيَ اللَّهُ الَّذِي نَزَّلَ الْكِتَابَ وَهُوَ يَتَوَلَّى الصَّالِحِينَ

> My Guardian is indeed God who sent down the Book, and He takes care of the righteous. (7:196)

By the sending of revelations and inspirations to the believers and the righteous, God takes them to the world-with-Allah, where they realise His presence and live the Goodly Life. And this is a solid path which no Muslim should miss - so that he can receive its true meaning from God Himself in the world-with-Allah. Of course, Satan also gathers friends by deceiving people using false revelations and temptations. Satan makes them attached to this world and thus prevents them from realising the world-with-Allah. He makes them blind to the truth and causes them to be his slaves, selling their divine pledge for a cheap price and making them forget their pledge which said:

$$\text{أَن لَّا تَعْبُدُوا الشَّيْطَانَ}$$

Do not worship Satan. (36:60)

Satan uses the methods that God uses for guiding man but for the opposite purpose. Revelation is one example:

$$\text{إِنَّ الشَّيَاطِينَ لَيُوحُونَ إِلَىٰ أَوْلِيَائِهِمْ}$$

Indeed, the satans inspire their friends. (6:121).

Another example can be the Qur'an itself, which is a source of guidance for believers, but a source of loss for oppressors.[41] This is why God has said to seek the protection of God against Satan when reciting the Qur'an. And this is not only by saying *"A'ūdh-u bi'llāh"* (I seek the protection of God) at the beginning of the recitation, but we should sincerely remember God throughout the recitation so that we can feel His guidance and protection and entrust ourselves to it.[42]

Protecting the Goodly Life

We previously mentioned that the Goodly Life actualizes in the world-with-Allah and with His mastership and also that the material earthly life is under the mastership of Satan. We should be careful not to allow Satan to gain influence with us and turn the Goodly Life into a life of corruption.

Satan can gain influence upon those who have not completely purified their hearts and are not completely obedient to Allah. But the true believers who have completely accepted Allah's mastership and obey Him in all aspects of their life have closed all the doors to Satan so that he can never gain any influence with them.

$$\text{إِنَّهُ لَيْسَ لَهُ سُلْطَانٌ عَلَى الَّذِينَ آمَنُوا وَعَلَىٰ رَبِّهِمْ يَتَوَكَّلُونَ}$$

Indeed, he does not have any authority over those who have faith and put their trust in their Lord. (16:99)

"Put their trust in their Lord" means they leave everything to their Lord[43] and trust in His mastership and guidance and this prepares them for the special supervision of Allah.

هُوَ مَوْلَانَا وَعَلَى اللهِ فَلْيَتَوَكَّلِ الْمُؤْمِنُونَ

He is our Master, and in God let all the faithful put their trust. (9:51)

وَاللهُ وَلِيُّهُمَا وَعَلَى اللهِ فَلْيَتَوَكَّلِ الْمُؤْمِنُونَ

God is their Guardian, and in God let all the faithful put their trust. (3:122)

إِنِّي تَوَكَّلْتُ عَلَى اللهِ رَبِّي وَرَبِّكُم مَّا مِن دَابَّةٍ إِلَّا هُوَ آخِذٌ بِنَاصِيَتِهَا

Indeed I have put my trust in God, my Lord and your Lord. There is no living being but He holds it by its forelock. (11:56)

Patience is the basis of the Goodly Life and trust is its protector. The same order can be understood from the following verse:

وَالَّذِينَ آمَنُوا وَعَمِلُوا الصَّالِحَاتِ لَنُبَوِّئَنَّهُم مِّنَ الْجَنَّةِ غُرَفًا تَجْرِي مِن تَحْتِهَا الْأَنْهَارُ خَالِدِينَ فِيهَا نِعْمَ أَجْرُ الْعَامِلِينَ الَّذِينَ صَبَرُوا وَعَلَىٰ رَبِّهِمْ يَتَوَكَّلُونَ

Those who have faith and do righteous deeds, We will surely settle them in lofty abodes of paradise with streams running in them, to remain in them [forever]. How excellent is the reward of the

workers! Those who exercised patience and put
their trust in their Lord. (29:58-59)

In this verse, after mentioning faith and righteous deeds - similar
to what is also mentioned in verse 16:97 about the Goodly Life -
the true condition of the people of paradise is described and its
everlasting quality is emphasised. In the Arabic version of this
verse, patience is mentioned in the past tense (i.e. *sabarū*) and
trust is mentioned in the present tense (i.e. *yatwakkalūn*). This
shows that patience is the basis of the Goodly Life and occurs
before its attainment, and putting trust in God is always
connected with the Goodly Life and is its protector. It may be
inferred from the verse that the difficulty of patience occurs
before the realization of the Goodly Life, and after the *fitri*
tendencies overcome the material temptations, the hardship of
patience has concluded. But putting trust in Allah is needed from
the beginning of moving towards the Goodly Life and fighting
with the *nafs* because patience needs a strong will and
determination and trusting Allah is needed in these matters. This
is also clear in the two following verses:

$$ إِن تَصْبِرُوا وَتَتَّقُوا فَإِنَّ ذَٰلِكَ مِنْ عَزْمِ الْأُمُورِ $$

If you are patient and God-conscious, that is indeed
the steadiest of courses. (3:186)

And in every act of determination, it is said to trust God:

$$ فَإِذَا عَزَمْتَ فَتَوَكَّلْ عَلَى اللَّهِ $$

And once you are resolved, put your trust in God.
(3:159)

Thus in order to succeed in the fight against the *nafs,* and to be
patient and persevere in this hard task, putting trust in God is
essential. In another verse of the Qur'an, putting trust in God is
mentioned as the link to the Divine life:

129

وَتَوَكَّلْ عَلَى الْحَيِّ الَّذِي لَا يَمُوتُ

Put your trust in the Living One who does not die.
(25:58)

This verse clearly shows that trust is the link to the divine life and
the support for the Goodly Life because, in the mystic point of
view, "an alive person is the one whose life is dependent on his
Creator's Life"[44] and this is in fact the Goodly Life. But physical
life does not depend on the divine life; it is dependent on God's
creatorship (khāliqiyyat) and sustainership (rāziqiyyat).

Warning and Action

إِنَّمَا سُلْطَانُهُ عَلَى الَّذِينَ يَتَوَلَّوْنَهُ وَالَّذِينَ هُم بِهِ مُشْرِكُونَ

His authority is only over those who befriend him
and those who make him a partner [of God].
(16:100)

Satan can only deceive the people who have accepted him as a
partner of God and act upon his temptations. In other words, they
commit polytheism due to their weak faith.

وَمَا يُؤْمِنُ أَكْثَرُهُم بِاللَّهِ إِلَّا وَهُم مُّشْرِكُونَ

And most of them do not believe in God without
ascribing partners to Him. (12:106)

Therefore, if Satan has authority upon us and we find difficulties
in performing righteous deeds, the only reason is that our lower
self (nafs) still remains influential and we are not absolutely
submissive to God. This is where Satan appears and tempts us by
creating a delusional world that captivates us.

Thus, we have to try to prepare for the presence in the world-
with-Allah and the actualisation of the Goodly Life. We have to
be patient and firm throughout the entire path of struggling with

130

our *nafs*. To succeed in this struggle, we have to get gradually closer to the divine Mastership and the Prophet and his Household and heed their call with our hearts, putting our trust in God.

$$\text{يَا أَيُّهَا الَّذِينَ آمَنُوا اسْتَجِيبُوا لِلَّهِ وَلِلرَّسُولِ إِذَا دَعَاكُمْ لِمَا يُحْيِيكُمْ}$$

> O you who have faith! Answer God and the Apostle when he summons you to that which will give you life. (8:24)

The Blaming Soul (*al-Nafs al-Lawwāmah*) can confront the Commanding Soul (*al-Nafs al-Ammārah*), but when the latter has Satan as its aid, we have to seek the protection of God's mastership to keep the balance in this combat so that the assistance of God might save us and include us in His special mercy.

Therefore, the realisation of the Goodly Life needs patience, trust in God, and consent to his mastership, all of which can be achieved by obedient believers through advancing in the levels of faith.

Finally we pray to God:

$$\text{و اجعلنى ممن ... احبيته حياة طيبة فى ادوم السرور و اسبغ الكرامة و اتمّ العيش}$$

> O my Lord, make me one of those you have revived to the Goodly Life in the most enduring happiness and the most perfect generosity and joy with no deficiency.[45]

131

[1] Fazl ibn Hasan ibn Tabarsi, *Majma' al-Bayān,* translated by Ali Karamy, (Tehran: Farahani, 1380 S.A.H.), vol. 7, pp. 734-735.

[2] Nasir Makarim Shirazi and others, *Tafsir-e Nemuneh,* vol. 13 (Qum: Dar al-Kutub al-Islami, 1373), vol. 11, p. 394.

[3] Abdullah Jawadi Amuli, *Fitrat dar Qur'an,* vol. 2 (Qum: Isrā', 1379), pp. 120-121.

[4] Muhammad Muhammadi Reyshahri, *Mizān al-Hikmah* (Qom, Dar al-Hadith, 1416 L.A.H.), vol. 3, Chapter: Ma'rifat (3), no. 12398, p. 1905.

[5] Ibid., p. 135.

[6] Sayyid Muhammad Husayn Tabataba'i, *Al-Mizan fi Tafsir al-Qur'an* (Beirut, Mu'assasat al-A'lami li'l-Matbu'āt, 1417 L.A.H.), vol. 8, p. 353.

[7] Hasan Mustafawi, *Al-Tahqiq fi Kalimāt al-Qur'an al-Karim* (Tehran: Ministry of Islamic Guidance, 1369 L.A.H.), vol. 11, p. 14.

[8] Sayyed Muhammad Husayn Tabataba'i, *Al-Mizān* (Beirut: Mu'assasat al-A'lami li'l-Matbu'āt, 1417 L.A.H.), vol. 16, p. 154

[9] Hasan Mustafawi, *Al-Tahqiq fi Kalimāt al-Qur'an al-Karim* (Tehran: Ministry of Islamic Guidance, 1369 L.A.H.), vol. 5, p. 274.

[10] Ibid., vol. 11, p. 188.

[11] Ibid., vol. 7, p. 207.

[12] Imam Khomeini, *Misbāh al-Hidāyah ila'l-Khilāfat-i wa'l-Wilāyah,* 2nd edition (Tehran, Mu'assesey-e Tanzim wa Nashr-e Athār-e Imam Khomeini, 1373 S.A.H.), p. 26; Sayyid Mahdi Bahr al-'Ulum, *Risāley-e Sayr-u Soluk,* with introduction and commentary by Muhammad Husayn Husayni Tehrani, 5th edition (Tehran: Nour-e Malakut-e Qur'an), p. 53; Abdullah Jawadi Amuli *Hayāt-i Haqiqiy-e Insān dar Qur'an* (Qum: Isrā', 1382 S.A.H.), pp. 238-248.

[13] Sayyid Muhammad Husayn Tabataba'i, *Al-Mizan* (Beirut: Mu'assasat al-A'lami li'l-Matbu'āt, 1417 L.A.H.), vol. 8, p. 327.

[14] Akbar Hashemi Rafsanjani, *Tafsir-e Rahnamā,* 2nd edition (Qum: Bustān-e Kitaā, 1380 S.A.H.), vol. 9, p. 525; Nasir Makarem Shirazi, *Tafsir-e Nemuneh,* 13th edition (Qum: Dar al-Kutub-e Islamiyyah, 1373 S.A.H.), vol. 11, p. 389.

[15] Muhammad Baqir Majlesi, *Bihār al-Anwār,* vol. 95, p. 363.

[16] The verse number 22 of *Surah al-Shura* mentions the same point.

[17] Refer to Sayyid Muhammad Husayn Tabataba'i, *Risālah al-Wilāyah,* appendix of the book *Tariq-e Irfan* (translation of *Risālah al-Wilāyah*),

translated by Sadiq Husaynzadeh (Qum: Bakhshayesh Publications, 1381 S.A.H.), p. 170, 190-191.

[18] Abdullah Jawadi Amuli, "Didgāhe 'Allamah dar Bāb-i Wilāyat-e Ilāhi," *Mirāth-e Javidan*, Second Issue (1369 S.A.H.), second year, p. 95.

[19] Qur'an 6:126; 7:26; 18:57; 32:22; 24:1; 40:3; 2:221; 21:42

[20] Hamid Reza Mazaheri Seif, "Nazariey-e Qur'an dar Bāb- i Chistiy-e 'Ilm," *Ma'rifat*, Issue 83 (Aban 1383 S.A.H.), p. 80.

[21] Muhammad ibn Ya'qub Kulayni, *Usul al-Kāfi*, vol. 1, p. 192, no. 2.

[22] Ibid., vol. 1, p. 194, no 1.

[23] Qur'an 9:22; 8:28; 64:15; etc.

[24] *Nahj al-Balāghah*, the Sermon 193 on the Pious (al-Muttaqin).

[25] "To God belongs the Unseen of the heavens and the earth. The matter of the Hour is just like the twinkling of an eye." (Qur'an 16:77)

[26] Muhammad Baqir Majlesi, *Bihār al-Anwār*, vol. 27, p. 24.

[27] *Nahj al-Balāghah*, Sermon no 203.

[28] Muhammad Baqir Majlesi, *Bihār al-Anwār*, vol. 4, p. 317.

[29] Ibid., vol. 70, p. 391.

[30] Qur'an (57:19)

[31] Muhammad Dashti, *Farhang- i Sukhanān- i Imam Husayn (a.s)* (Qum: Mu'assese-ye Tahqiqāti-ye Amir al-Mu'menin (as), 1377 S.A.H.), p. 579.

[32] Abdullah Jawadi Amuli, *Tahrir-i Tamhid al-Qawā'id* (Tehran: Al-Zahra, 1372 S.A.H.), p. 3.

[33] Muhammad Taqi Misbah Yazdi, *Akhlaq dar Qur'an* (Qum: Imam Khomeini Education & Research Institute), vol. 1, pp. 128-130.

[34] Refer to Mulla Sadra, *Sharh Usul al-Kāfi*.

[35] Muhammad Baqir Majlesi, *Bihār al-Anwār*, vol. 53, p. 191.

[36] Sayyed Muhammad Husayn Tabataba'i, *Al-Mizan* (Beirut: Mu'assasat al-A'lami li'l-Matbu'āt, 1417 L.A.H.), vol. 1, pp. 195-198

[37] Refer to Nasir Makarem Shirazi, *Ayāt-e Wilāyat dar Qur'an* (Qum, Nasl-e Javān, 1381 S.A.H.), p. 81.

[38] Muhammad Baqir Majlesi, *Bihār al-Anwār*, vol. 36, p. 13, no. 19.

[39] Ibid., pp. 13-14.

[40] Sayyed Muhammad Husayn Tabataba'i, *Al-Mizān* (Beirut: Mu'assasat al-A'lami lil-Matbu'āt, 1417 L.A.H.), vol. 7, p. 348.

[41] Qur'an 17:82.

[42] Ibid., vol. 12, p. 348.

[43] Refer to Hasan Mustafawi, *Al-Tahqiq fī Kalimāt al-Qur'an al-Karim* (Tehran, Ministry of Islamic Guidance, 1369 L.A.H.), vol. 13, p. 193.

[44] Sayyed Sadiq Goharin, *Sharh-i Istilāhāt-i Tasawwuf* (Tehran: Zuwwār, 1368 S.A.H.), vol. 4, p. 314.

[45] Muhammad Baqir Majlesi, *Bihār al-Anwār*, vol. 95, p. 91.

Respect for Animal Life in Islam

Ali Ahmadi Khah

Abstract

The Prophet Muhammad (s), has given rules and regulations for the rights of all living creatures, including humans and animals. These rules and regulations, which were introduced 1400 years ago, show the attentiveness of Islam towards the rights of all living creatures. In this article, animal rights will be explored from the perspective of Prophet Muhammad (s). One of the conclusions of this article is that, when the Holy Prophet (s) afforded so much attention to the rights of animals, he had most certainly paid attention to human rights as well.

It has to be made explicit here that, when we say that animals have rights in Islam, there are also a set of responsibilities which have to be accepted by human beings. This means that if humans do not respect the rights of animals, they are sinners and will be punished on the Day of Judgement. In some cases, these sinners will be questioned in this world as well. For example, in conformity with Shi'a Islamic jurisprudence, in any case in which the owner of an animal does not fulfil its needs, the ruler has to force the owner to fulfil these needs, and if the owner is incapable of doing so, it is the responsibility of other people to fulfil these needs and maintain the life of the animal.

Islamic thought is based on the book (the Holy Qur'an) and the tradition (the sayings and actions) of the Prophet. In Islamic system of thought, there is a great deal of reinforcement for the importance of the life of living creatures and providing for their needs. The Most Glorious God has Himself taken on the responsibility of providing sustenance, and in the Holy Qur'an, He has considered everything that moves, including birds and all grazing animals, to be communities similar to the community of human beings. Thus it is said:

وَ ما مِنْ دَابَّةٍ فِى الْأَرْضِ وَ لا طائِرٍ يَطيرُ بِجَناحَيْهِ إِلاَّ أُمَمٌ أَمْثالُكُمْ ما فَرَّطْنا فِى الْكِتابِ مِنْ شَىْءٍ ثُمَّ إِلى رَبِّهِمْ يُحْشَرُونَ

There is no animal on land, nor a bird that flies with its wings, but they are communities like yourselves. We have not omitted anything from the Book. Then they will be gathered toward their Lord. (6:38)

In another verse, the Qur'an has talked about providing for the urgent needs and necessities of life for animals and has placed them next to those of humans:

وَ كَأَيِّنْ مِنْ دَابَّةٍ لا تَحْمِلُ رِزْقَهَا اللّهُ يَرْزُقُها وَ إِيّاكُمْ وَ هُوَ السَّميعُ الْعَليمُ

How many an animal there is that does not carry its own provision. God provides for it, and for you, and He is the All-hearing, the All-knowing. (29:60)

The Qur'an considers any type of cruelty to animals, like cutting off their ears or tail, etc., as wrong and Satanic:

وَ لَأُضِلَّنَّهُمْ وَ لَأُمَنِّيَنَّهُمْ وَ لَآمُرَنَّهُمْ فَلَيُبَتِّكُنَّ آذانَ الْأَنْعامِ وَ لَآمُرَنَّهُمْ فَلَيُغَيِّرُنَّ خَلْقَ اللّهِ وَ مَنْ يَتَّخِذِ الشَّيْطانَ وَلِيًّا مِنْ دُونِ اللّهِ فَقَدْ خَسِرَ خُسْراناً مُبيناً

And I [Satan] will lead them astray and give them [false] hopes, and prompt them to slit the ears of cattle, and I will prompt them to alter God's creation. Whoever takes Satan as a guardian instead of God has certainly incurred a manifest loss. (4:119)

In these three verses, three important and essential points have been considered:

Firstly, all living creatures have a social community. Of course, because of the natural differences between humans and animals, these communities have different social structures. Yet regardless of these differences, animals still have their own communities. Secondly, the providing of sustenance for both animals and humans is undertaken by God, and thus it is said: *God provides for it and for you.* Therefore, God's book, which is the eternal miracle of the Holy Prophet (s), pays special attention to the essential needs of animals, to the extent that it has placed them alongside the needs of humans; Thirdly, the amputation of the limbs of animals is considered Satanic and hurting and misusing animals is called a Satanic action; indeed, it has been referred to as a great loss.[1]

The Protection of Animals

In addition to the Qur'an, we find many instructions concerning the rights of animals in the sayings and actions of the Holy Prophet (s). For example, the Prophet Muhammad is quoted as saying:

مَنْ قَتَلَ عصفوراً عبثاً، جاء يوم القيامة يعجّ الى الله تعالى يقول: يا ربّ انَّ هذا قَتَلَنى عَبَثاً لَمْ يُنْتَفَعْ بى و لم يدعنى فآكل مِنْ حشارة الأرض

If someone kills a robin in vein, it will shout in the presence of Allah on the Day of Judgement and say: This person killed me without even getting

137

any profit out of this killing! And he did not let me use the insects on earth and feed on them.[2]

ما من انسان يقتل عصفوراً فما فوقها بغير حقّها الا سأله الله عنها. قيل يا رسول الله و ما حقّها؟ قال: أن يذبحها فيأكلها و أن لا يقطع رأسها و يرمى به

If anyone kills a robin or a bigger one without respecting its rights, God Almighty will interrogate them on the Day of Judgement. It was asked, 'Oh Holy Prophet! What are the rights of a robin?' He replied: 'That it is slaughtered according to Islamic rules, not that its neck is just ripped off.'[3]

ما من دابّة طائر و لا غيره يُقْتَلُ بغير الحقّ الا ستُخاصِمُه يَومَ القيامة

If any animal or bird is killed unjustifiably or not, it will appeal against its murderer on the Day of Judgement.[4]

Imam Musa ibn Jafar (a) has quoted from his honoured fathers (a) that the Holy Prophet (s) has stated:

و رأيت فى النار صاحبة الهرّة تنهشها مقبلةً و مدبرةً، كانت أوثقها لم تكن تطعمها و لم ترسلها تأكل من حشاش الارض

I saw a woman in hell whose cat was biting her everywhere; The reason was because this women had tied up this animal on earth, without giving it any food or setting it free to eat.[5]

In another narration, he spoke about the women's harsh punishment:

A woman was rightly put in the flames of hell and was punished for her treatment of a cat, as she had tied up the cat and did not let it free to find food for itself and because of this the cat had starved to death. [6]

Ibn Abbas says that the Holy Prophet (s) has said not to kill any living creature unless it brings harm. [7]

The Prophet not only prohibited the killing of living creatures, but ordered the believers to be careful at night so that a small creature or small insect would not be stepped on, even inadvertently.

> When a division of the night has passed, try to go out less, as there are God's creatures which he will spread out on the earth at those hours. [8]

Anas ibn Malik (one of the companions of the Prophet) said that the Holy Prophet (s) has said: *"Do not kill ants!"* [9] Also, in a trustworthy narration, the Prophet prohibited eating what an ant carries by its mouth and legs. [10]

Malik ibn Anas reports that the Prophet (s) did not like to destroy their nests by burning them. [11] In general, we find that the Prophet of compassion has prohibited the hurting and torturing of animals using fire and has said in this regard:

$$ لا يعذب بالنار الا الله تعالى $$

> No one, except God, can use fire to hurt and punish anyone else. [12]

Therefore burning animals with fire is not allowed.

According to a both Nisa'i and Ahmad, a physician discussed the use of frogs in medicine with the Prophet (s). The Prophet immediately banned the doctor from killing frogs. [13]

The Prophet did not like hunting either and said: *"Whoever gets involved in hunting will forget things relevant to the afterlife."* [14]

According to another narration, it is also mentioned that the Prophet (s) never went hunting and never recommended that Muslims perform this action.[15] There is another narration which states that the Prophet Muhammad (s) ordered Muslims not to hurt (i.e., kill) animals unless it is for eating their meat[16] (with the caveat that the meat is Halal and therefore allowed by Islamic teachings).

Shaddad ibn Aws says that the Prophet of Islam (s) said: *"God has involved kindness in everything; if you want to kill an animal for food, kill it nicely, make the knife sharp and take the animal out of its agony as fast as possible."*[17] The Prophet of kindness (s) saw a person who had laid down a sheep, and while he was sharpening his knife, had his leg on the sheep's throat while the sheep was looking at him. The Prophet (s) said to him: *"Do you want to slaughter it according to Islamic rules or kill it twice?"*[18]

When the Prophet of Islam saw an Arab who was beating sheep with his cane, he said: *"Bring him, but don't scare him."* When they brought him, he told the man: *"Don't beat the sheep with your cane, but move them about with kindness and gentleness."*[19]

Once, someone wanted to catch his animal, and as the animal was used to coming to him when he was shown a bowl, or the skirt of his owner, which represented the feeding of barley or salt, the owner, who didn't have any barley or salt with him, tricked the animal using this same method and caught it. The Holy Prophet (s), who was watching this scene, got upset and said: *"Why did you lie to this animal, you shouldn't have tricked it!"*[20]

In one of the wars, the wife of one of the *Ansar* (a group of Muslims who lived in the city of Medina and helped the Muslim immigrants coming from Mecca) was held hostage and managed to escape with one of the camels of the Prophet (s) from the area in which she was imprisoned; when she arrived in Madinah and went to the Prophet (s), she said: "I had a *nadhr* (to promise to do a certain act if a certain event happens) that if I was saved I would sacrifice the camel." The Prophet said:

What a bad prize you have given the camel, it has carried you and saved you, and then you want to kill it?! You should know that nadhr is not right and is discarded when there is sin in it or if you are not the owner of that animal.[21]

Imam Musa ibn Ja'far narrates from his respectable fathers (a) that the Holy Prophet (s) was passing a group of people. The group had tied up a baby chicken somewhere high up and were shooting it using a bow and arrow! When the Prophet (s) saw this scene, he said: *Who are these people?! May god curse them!*[22]

The Prophet (s) not only did not approve of imprisoning human beings but did not like imprisoning animals. He has said:

> There isn't a family who ties up and keeps a dog (imprisoned), whose good deeds doesn't decrease slightly each day, except for a hurtful dog, hunting dog, guard dog for farming or guarding sheep... (and according to another narration) and a dog guarding a house.[23]

It should not be left unsaid, however, that killing animals which cause harm to human beings is allowed; one such animal is a rabid dog. However, in the view of Islam, even in these cases, it is not lawful to imprison them so that they die of starvation and dehydration, but they must be killed in specific ways. Another point that must be made is that, in Islam, killing dogs has a penalty that has to be paid (*diyah*). The fine for killing a hunting dog is forty dirhams and the fine for killing a guard dog is twenty dirhams.[24]

According to historians, when the Prophet (s) was travelling with the Muslim army to triumph over the victory at Makkah, he saw a dog that was howling at her kids while they were feeding from her. He told Ju'ayl ibn Suraqah to stand by the dog and take care of her so that when the army was passing they wouldn't harm the dog and her puppies.[25]

141

The Curse on Those who Amputate Animals

The Prophet (s) did not even like cutting an animal's tails and ears, let alone castrating or killing them! According to a narration, the Holy Prophet (s) said: *"May God curse those who amputate animals."*[26] In another narration, he ordered the Muslims not to castrate horses.[27]

The Reward of Kindness to Animals

The Prophet Muhammad (s) is quoted as saying:

> A sinful woman saw a thirsty dog who was standing above a well panting. He would soon have died of thirst if the woman hadn't intervened. The woman took her shoe off, tied it to her scarf and used it to pull water out of the well and gave it to the dog. God forgave her sins for her kindness to this animal.[28]

According to another narration, the Prophet has said:

> A thirsty woman was passing by when she saw a well. She went into it, drank some, and came out. She saw a dog panting next to the well. She said to herself: 'This dog is feeling like I did when I was thirsty.' She went back into the well, filled her shoe with water and held it to the dog's mouth until he was hydrated. God forgave her sins for this action."

In another narration, it's been said that it was asked from Prophet Muhammad (s) if being kind to animals has any reward, he said:

> Yes, for every thirsty being that you hydrate, there is a reward.[29]

It has been written that when the Prophet (s) was performing *wudhu* (ritual ablution), a cat approached him. The Prophet (s) knew that the animal was thirsty so he pushed the container of water towards it and the cat drank. Then he performed *wudhu*.[30]

Ban from Milking All the Milk of Animals

The Prophet (s) has said that supporting any living thing has a reward from God, and he has emphasised not to milk animals too much, to leave milk for their young ones, to place saddles in the right place, not to put anything sharp near or in an animal's mouth, not to overload them with things to carry and always keep the animal where it can be dry.[31]

One of the followers of the Prophet of Islam (s) said: The Prophet (s) liked sheep. One day a sheep entered the house and took a loaf of bread near us and ran away. I got up quickly and ran after it and removed the bread from its mouth. When the Prophet (s) saw this, he said:

> That wasn't a nice thing you did; it wasn't right for you to hold the animal from the back of its neck and pressurise it so that you could get the bread![32]

One of the companions of the Holy Prophet (s) said: A lactating camel was given to the Prophet as a present. He told me to milk it. I milked it as much as I could. When the Prophet saw the extent to which I was milking it, he said: *"Do not milk it that way! Leave some for its children.*[33]

Ban from Hunting Birds at Night Time

One saying from the Prophet regarding this issue is:

> Don't take baby chickens out of their nests at night time, and don't take birds out of their nests to be killed when it's time for them to sleep but wait until morning.

A man asked, "What do you mean when it's time for them to sleep?" The Prophet answered:

143

Night time is time for them to sleep. Therefore do not disturb them at night until morning. And also do not remove and kill the children of birds which don't have feathers yet and can't fly! Let them reach the age where they can fly and then you can hunt them.[34]

The Holy Prophet (s) said:

Amongst the previous nations, a man had found a bird nest and whenever the bird had baby chickens, he removed them and took them with him. That bird complained to God of what had happened. Through a revelation, God told the bird that if that man comes back again, I will kill him.[35]

Ibn Mas'ud said: We were with the Prophet when a man entered the jungle carrying an egg he had taken from the nest of a bird. The bird followed us, flying in circles around us, and was very disturbed. When the Prophet saw this scene, he said: Which one of you has disturbed and stricken this bird? The man said: I have taken the egg or the baby chicken of the bird. The Prophet said: *Have mercy upon her and return the egg to her! Return it to her!*"[36] Also, at the same time, he saw that an ant's nest was set on fire, he said:

Who has set this nest on fire? It is not acceptable that anyone uses fire in the means of torture, except the God of fire.[37]

In another narration, 'Āmir al-Rām says: We were sitting in the presence of the Prophet (s) when a man entered wearing a cloak. He was holding something which he had wrapped at the corner of his cloak. The man said: "Oh Prophet of God! When I saw you from afar, I came towards you. On the way I passed some trees when I heard the sound of some baby chickens. I went and caught them and put them in my cloak. When I did this, their mother came and circled around my head; I opened my cloak for her and she came down upon her baby chickens, so I wrapped my cloak and brought them all together." The Prophet said: *"Put them on the ground!"* I placed them on the ground, but I saw that the mother would not leave her baby chickens and run away! The Prophet said: *"Are you surprised at the kindness of the mother of the baby chickens for her young?"* They said: "Yes!" He said: *"I swear upon the one who made me Prophet, God is more kind towards his slaves than this bird towards her baby chickens! You, man, return them to where you found them!"* And I returned them.[38]

Rights of Riding Animals

In a reliable narration, it has been said that there are certain rights for riding animals that their owners must respect. For instance, when you obtain an animal, you have to give it food; if you pass a place with water, wait, and show the water to the animal; do not hit the face of an animal, as it worships God; do not use its back as a place to rest upon or talk; do not make an animal carry anything more than it is able; and do not ride it more than it is able.[39] According to a narration by Anas, the Prophet (s) said:

> It is crucial for the owner of the riding animal to respect the spirit in the animal and feed it and give it water.[40]

It has also been said that the Prophet of Islam (s) had mentioned horses, and said:

> Great good is attached to the forelocks of horses even till the day of judgment, and whoever does them any good for God's sake, will have the reward of a person whose hands are never drawn back for giving charity; ready hands for giving charity that are not drawn back.[41]

The Prophet of kindness (s) said:

> Do not cut short the forelocks of horses, as there is good in it. Do not cut their mane as it keeps them

warm.[42] Do not cut or shorten their tail as they use it to ward off insects and flies.[43]

And he also said:

قال رسول الله (ص): ان الله و ملائكته يصلّون على
أصحاب الخيل...

God and his angels bless those who own horses.[44]

According to another narration, the Prophet has said:

عن على (ع) قال: أنّ رسول الله (ص) قال: الخيل معقود
بنواصيها الخير الى يوم القيامة؛ و من ارتبط فرساً فى
السبيل الله كان علفه و روثه و شرابه فى ميزانه يوم
القيامة

Whoever takes a horse to its stable, with intentions to please God, feeds it, gives it water and cleans its stable; this will all be taken into account on the Day of Judgment and will be awarded.[45]

Tamim Dārimi was seen cleaning his horse's barley. The people asked him, "Why don't you let someone else do this for you?" He said I heard the Prophet of Islam (s) say:

There isn't a man who cleans his horse's barley and doesn't get a good deed written for him for every grain he has cleaned.[46]

Respecting the Rights of Animals While Riding or Using Them to Carry Things

As we have said before, Prophet Muhammad (s) has given certain orders which value riding animals, such as being kind to them, not making them walk or run faster than their ability, not putting goods on them which are heavier than they can carry, not making them travel on routes which are difficult to pass, not riding them uphill, not sitting on them to talk to people or using them as a seat, letting them benefit from grass fields, not keeping them in deserted places, providing them with water and grass throughout journeys and after arriving at designated destinations. In what follows, we will further introduce Prophet Muhammad's (s) orders in this regard.

The Prophet (s) has said to all who ride animals that, while riding upon them, do not sit on them in a way which will hurts them and do not use them as your seats;[47] meaning when the animal is not moving do not remain seated on them while speaking to others, rather come down and speak. Another time, he said:

> Do not use animals as your chair when you want to speak to someone in the street since there may be many animals that are better than their riders and invoke God more.[48]

Prophet Muhammad (s) used to say all the time:

> Do not use animals as chairs and pulpits when you want to give a speech. Animals have been created by God to take you to your destination through ways that are hard for you to pass. [Come down and] speak to each other on the ground.[49]

In another place, he also said:

> Regarding animals that are not able to defend themselves, you have to be afraid of God's punishment; while riding them, sit on them properly. If you want to eat those of them which are allowed, slaughter them as ordered and then eat them properly. And choose the fat ones to eat.[50]

On how to ride animals, he has said:

اذا رَكِبَ أحدُكم الدابّةَ، فليحملها على ملاذّها

Whenever one of you is riding an animal, he has to take it on paths which are smooth and easy to pass while avoiding the difficult ones.[51]

In another place, he said:

من مشى عن راحلته عُقَبَةً، فكأنما أعتق رقبةً

Whoever comes down off his animal uphill and walks behind it, is like someone who has liberated a slave for the sake of God.[52]

Jabir narrates that the Prophet (s) used to prohibit the riding of three people on an animal.[53] A similar admonition can be seen in one of his other statements, where he says:

لا يرتدف ثلثة على دابة؛ فان أحدهم ملعون و هو مقدّم

Not more than two people are allowed to ride an animal, otherwise one of them will be cursed - the one in front.[54]

Furthermore, regarding using animals to carry things, he said:

أخرّوا الأحمال فانّ اليدين معلّقة و الرجلين موثّقة

Put the goods on the backside, because if you put it in front, the animal cannot walk properly due to the close distance of the goods to its hands which will prevent moving when the goods are heavy and also because of the hardness of their legs.[55]

About respecting animals during a journey, the Prophet of kindness (s) said:

اذا سِرتم فى أرض خصبة فأعطوا الدوابَّ حظَّها و ان
سرتم فى أرض مُدبة فانجوا عليها؛ و اذا عرَّستم فلا
تعرسوا على القارعة الطريق، فانّها مأوى كل دابة

When passing a green land that has grass, let your
camels benefit from the land (let them pasture and
eat and become satisfied) but when passing a
deserted land, do not stop and get to a green land
quick.[56]

Regarding kindness and tolerance with animals, the Prophet (s) said:

ان الله تبارك و تعالى يُحبُّ الرِّفْقَ وَ يُعينُ عليه. فاذا
رَكِبْتُمْ الدَّوابَّ الْعِجافَ فأنْزِلوها مَنازِلَها؛ فانْ كانَت
الأرضُ مُجْدِبَةً فانْجوا عليها و انْ كانتْ مُخْصِبَةً فأنزِلوها
منازِلَها

God likes kindness and will help to put it into
practice. Therefore, whenever you ride an animal
take him to its place afterwards, while passing a
bare and deserted land with them, cross it quickly
and while passing a green land, let them rest there.
57

He also said:

من سافر منكم بدابة، فاليبدء حين ينزل بعلفها و سقيها

Whenever you have travelled while riding an
animal, the first thing you should do after getting
down is to give them water and feed them with
grass.[58]

There is another statement from the Prophet (s) which shows the
great mercy and compassion he had:

لو غُفِرَ لكم ما تأتون الى البهائم، لَغُفِرَ لكم كثيراً

149

If you get forgiven for what you have done to animals, indeed a great deal of your sins will be forgiven.[59]

Once the Prophet (s) was passing somewhere and saw a camel tied to the doorknob of a house and having no grass or water to benefit from. The Prophet of mercy (s) said:

أين صاحب هذه الراحلة؟ ألا تتقى اللهَ فيها؟ اما أن تعلِفَها و اما أن ترسلَها؛ حتى تبتغى لنفسها

Where is the owner of this animal? Are not you afraid of God's punishment for what you have done to this animal? Either provide him with grass and water or let him free so that he can find food for himself.[60]

Prohibition of Cauterizing Animals and Making Them Fight Each Other

The Prophet (s) also has made recommendations and given guidance which prohibits cauterising animals and making them fight each other or carrying goods upon their bodies in a way which is harmful to them. The following are instances of his recommendations. Ibn Abbas narrates that the Prophet (s) prohibited making animals and birds fight each other as people used to make rams and roosters fight each other.[61] Another time he said:

ان الله تعالى لعن من يحرش بين البهائم

God curses those who make animals fight each other.[62]

In many narrations, Prophet Muhammad (s), the Prophet of mercy, has prohibited cauterising animals' faces.[63] He said:

Do not hit animals in their face, for every creature is in a state of praising God. Do not cauterise their faces, for there might be many animals that are better than their riders and obey God more and invoke God (more than those riding them).[64]

One time one of Hakam ibn Harith's camels would not stand on its legs and Hakam was beating the camel. The Prophet (s) told him: *"Do not beat it."* And then he told the camel: *"Hol Hol"* and the camel stood up on his legs.[65]

Once Sawādah ibn al-Rabi' went to Prophet Muhammad (s). The Prophet (s) gave him some camels and said:

> When you go back to your family, tell them to feed animals and to cut their nails so that while milking them, they won't scratch and wound their breast.[66]

Conclusion

What we have mentioned in this article about the manners and words of the Prophet (s) in relation to the caring for animals is only a part of his mercy and compassion towards animals. The Prophet of mercy (s) said even burning a termites nest or killing a frog will be punished. How then could such a person want mankind to be harmed or killed? Never. This was not his character.

Bibliography

The Holy Qur'an.

Nahj al-Balāghah.

Ahsā'i, Abi Jumhur, *'Awāli al-La'āli al-'Aziziyyah fi al-Ahādith al-Diniyyah*, revised by Sayyed Mar'ashi and Shaykh Mujtaba 'Araqi, 1st edition (Qum: Sayyed al-Shuhada Publications, 1403 L.A.H.).

Bayhaqi, Ahmad, *Al-Sunan al-Kubrā* (Beirut: Dār al-Fikr Publications).

Bukhari, Muhammad bin Isma'il, *Sahih Bukhari* (Beirut: Dār al-Fikr Publications).

Dumayri, Shaykh Kamal al-Din, *Hayāt al-Haywān al-Kubrā* (Beirut: Dār al-Fikr Publications).

Harrāni, Abi Muhammad Hasan, *Tuhaf al-'Uqul 'an Āl al-Rasul,* translated by Muhammad Baqir Kamare'i, revised and annotated by Ali Akbar Ghaffari, 7th edition (Tehran: Ketabchi Publications, 1379 S.A.H.).

Haythami, Nour al-Din, *Majma' al-Zawā'id wa Manba' al-Fawā'id* (Beirut: Dār al-Kutub al-'Ilmiyyah, 1408 L.A.H.).

Hurr al-'Amili, Shaykh Muhammad, *Wasāil al-Shi'a* (Beirut: Dār Ihyā' al-Turāth).

Hurr al-'Amili, Shaykh Muhammad, *Wasāil al-Shi'a*, 2nd edition (Qum: Mehr Publications, Mu'assasat Āl al-Bayt, 1414 L.A.H.).

Hurr al-Amili, Shaykh Muhammad, *Al-Fusul al-Muhimmah fi Usul il-A'immah,* revised by Muhammad Qai'ini, 1st edition (Qum: Mu'assiseh Ma'ārif Islami-ye Imam Rida (a), 1418 L.A.H.).

Ibn Athir, *Usd al-Ghābah* (Tehran: Isma'ilian Publications).

Ibn Hanbal, Ahmad, *Musnad* (Beirut: Dār al-Sadir Publications).

Ibn Sa'd, Muhammad, *Al-Tabāqāt al-Kubrā* (Beirut: Dār al-Sadir Publications).

Jabal 'Amili, Shahid Zayn al-Din, *Al-Rawdat al-Bahiyyah fi Sharh al-Lum'at al-Dimashqiyyah*, 7th edition (Qum: Islamic Propagation Office, 1372 S.A.H.).

Jawziyyah, Shams al-Din Muhammad, *Al-Tibb al-Nabawi* (Beirut: Dār al-Wifāq).

Katani, Sayyid Muhammad Abd al-Hayy, *Nizām al-Hukumat al-Nabawiyyah (al-Musammā al-Tarātib al-Idāriyyah)*, revised by Abdullah Khalidi, 2nd edition (Beirut: Sharikat Dār al-Arqam).

Majlesi, Muhammad Baqir, *Bihār al-Anwār,* 2nd edition (Beirut: Mu'assasat al-Wafā', 1403 L.A.H.).

Muhammadi Reyhshahri, Mohammad, *Mizān al-Hikmah,* translated by Hamid Reza Shaykhi, 2nd edition (Qum: Dār al-Hadith Publications, 1379 S.A.H.).

Muttaqi Hindy, 'Alā al-Din, *Kanz al-'Ummāl* (Beirut, Mu'assasat al-Risālah, 1409 L.A.H.).

Noury, Husayn, "Jāmi'iyyat-i Islam," in *Khātam-e Payāmbarān* (Tehran: Husayniyyah Irshad, 1348 S.A.H.).

Saduq, Muhammad ibn Ali ibn Babiwayh Qummi, *Al-Muqli'ah* (Qum: Al-Hādi Publications, 1415 L.A.H.).

Salehi Shami, Muhammad bin Yusuf, *Subul al-Rashād fi Sirat Khayr al-'Ibād,* revised by Shaykh 'Adil Ahmad Abd al-Mawjud, 1st edition (Beirut: Dar al-Kutub al-'Ilmiyyah, 1414 L.A.H.).

---

[1] To understand these verses better, please refer to *Al-Mizān fi Tafsir al-Qur'an by* 'Allamah Tabataba'i.

[2] *Bihār al-Anwār*, vol. 64, p. 4; vol. 61, pp. 270 and 306; *Mizān al-Hikmah*, vol. 3, p. 1348, hadith no. 4537.

[3] *Bihār al-Anwār*, vol. 64, p. 306.

[4] *Mizān al-Hikmah*, vol. 3, p. 1346, hadith no. 4536.

[5] *Bihār al-Anwār*, vol. 64, p. 268; vol. 65, p. 65; *Mizān al-Hikmah*, vol. 3, p. 1346, hadith no. 4533.

[6] *Mizān al-Hikmah*, vol. 3, p. 1346, hadith no. 4533.

[7] Ibid., hadith no. 4539.

[8] *Taysir al-Wusul ilā Jami' al-Usul*, vol. 4, p. 388, cited in *Khātam al-Nabiyyin*, p. 487.

[9] *Bihār al-Anwār*, vol. 64, pp. 244 and 291.

[10] Ibid., p. 261.

[11] *Hayāt al-Haywān al-Kubrā* by Kamāl al-Din Dumayri, vol. 2, p. 10.

[12] *Bihār al-Anwār*, vol. 64, p. 244; *Man Lā Yahduruhu al-Faqih*, vol. 4, p. 3.

[13] *Al-Tibb al-Nabawi* by Shams al-Din Muhammad Jawziyyah, pp. 122 and 259:

أن طبيباً ذكر ضِفْدعاً فى دواء عند رسول الله (ص) نهى رسول الله، عن قتلها.

It has been suggested that whoever eats the flesh or blood of frog for treatment or any other reason his body will swallow, his colour will change and his semen goes out without his will till he finally dies. Therefore, the physicians have banned its usage. (Ibid., pp. 259-260)

[14] *Bihār al-Anwār*, vol. 65, p. 281, no. 29.

[15] Sha'rani, *Manh ul-Minnah fi Talabbus bi'l-Sunnah*, p. 33, cited in Sayyid Muhammad Hayy al-Katani, *Nizām al-Hukumah an-Nabawiyyah (al-Musammā at-Tarātib al-Idāriyyah)*, revised by Abdullah Khaledi, vol. 2, p. 66.

[16] *Hayāt al-Haywān al-Kubrā*, Ibid., vol. 2, p. 363:

نهى (صلى الله عليه وآله) عن تعذيب الحيوان الاّ لمأكله

[17] *Bihār al-Anwār*, vol. 65, p. 315:

ان الله كتب عليكم الاحسان فى كل شىء؛ فاذا قتلتم، فأحسنوا القتلة؛ و اذا ذبحتم، فأحسنوا الذبحة وليحدّ أحدكم شفرته و ليرح ذبيحته

and it also says:

نهى النبى (ص) عن ذبح الحيوان الا لأكله

"In another narration, the prophet banned hunting animals unless it is with the intention of eating them." (Ibid., vol. 64, p. 8)

[18] Nour al-Din Haythami, *Majma'al-Zawā'id wa Manba' al-Fawā'id*, vol. 4, p. 33:

عن بن عباس، انه قال: مرّ رسول الله (ص) على رجل واضع
رجله على صفحة شاة و هو يحد شفرته و هى تلحظ اليه يبصرها.
قال (ص) أفلا قتل هذا أو يريد أن يميتها موتتين

[19] Ibn Athir, *Usd al-Ghābah*, vol. 1, p. 336, cited in *Khātam al-Nabiyyin*, p. 485.

20 Jawadi Amuli, cited in the website Baztab (the Month of Dey of 1384 S.A.H.).

21 Ahmad Bayhaqi, Sunan al-Kubrā, vol. 10, p. 75.

22 Nawādir by Ravandi, p. 43, cited in Bihār al-Anwār, vol. 64, p. 268, no. 30:

موسى بن جعفر عن آبائه (ع) قال: مرّ رسول الله (ص) على قوم
نصبوا دجاجةً حيةً و هم يرمونها بالنبل؛ فقال: من هؤلاء (!؟)
لعنهم الله!

[23] *Sahih Bukhari*, vol. 3, p. 67; *Musnad* of Ahmad ibn Hanbal, vol. 2, pp. 8, 37, 60, 101, 113, ...; *'Awāli al-La'āli*, vol. 3, p. 452.

[24] Refer to Shaykh Saduq, *Al-Muqni'ah*, p. 534.

[25] Muhammad ibn Yusuf Salih Shami, *Subul al-Rashād fi Sirat-e Khayr al-'Ibād*, vol. 5, p. 212 and vol. 7, p. 29:

لما سار رسول الله (ص)...نظر الى كلبة تهر عن اولادها و هن
حولها و يرضعنها، فأمر جُعَيل بن سراقة أن يقوم حذاءها فلا
يعرض لها أحد من الجيش و لا لأولادها

[26] *Kanz al-'Ummāl*, Ibid., vol. 9, p. 66, no. 24971, cited in *Mizān al-Hikmah*, vol. 3, p. 1344, no. 4522:

قال (ص): لعن اللهُ مَن مثّل بالحيوان

And also:

قال (ص): لعن اللهُ مَن يُمَثِّلُ بالبَهائم

"May God curse the one who castrates animals." (Ibid., vol. 9, p. 67, no. 24985)

[27] Ibid., vol. 9, p. 66, no. 24977:

نهى (ص) عن خِصاء الخيل و البهائم

[28] *Mizān al-Hikmah*, vol. 3, p. 1346, no. 4532; *Hayāt al-Haywān al-Kubrā*, Ibid., vol. 2, p. 378; *Jawāhir al-Kalām*, vol. 31, p. 359; *Bihār al-Anwār*, Ibid., vol. 65, p. 65, under the hadith number 24.

[29] *Hayāt al-Haywān al-Kubrā*, vol. 2 p. 378; *Bihār al-Anwār*, vol. 65, p. 65, under hadith number 24; *Mizān al-Hikmah*, vol. 3, p. 1346, no . 4532; Najafi, *Jawāhir al-Kalām,* vol. 31, p. 359:

روى مسلم أن النبى (ص) قال: بينما امرأة تمشى بفلاة من الأرض اشتد عليها العطش فنزلت بئر فشربت ثم صعدت فوجدت كلباً يأكل الثرى من العطش؛ فقالت لقد بلغ بهذا الكلب مثل الذى بلغ بى! ثم نزلت البئر، فملأت خفها و أمسكها بفيها ثم صعدت فسقته؛ فشكر الله لها ذالك و غفر لها. قالوا: يا رسول الله أ وَ لنا فى البهائم أجر؟ قال (ص): نعم فى كل كبد رطبة أجر.

[30] *Hayāt al-Haywān al-Kubrā*, vol. 2, p. 384; *Bihār al-Anwār*, vol. 16, p. 293. no. 160:

قال على (ع) : بينا رسول الله (ص) يتوضأ اذ لاذبه هرّ البيت، و عرف رسول الله (ص) أنه عطشان؛ فأصغى اليه الاناء حتى شرب منه الهرّ و توضأ بفضله

[31] *Nizām al-Hukumat al-Nabawiyyah,* vol. 2, p. 155, cited in *Khātam al-Nabiyyin,* p. 483.

[32] *Hayāt al-Haywān al-Kubrā*, vol. 2, p. 44:

فدخلت شاة فأخذت قرصاً تحت دن لنا، فقمت اليها فأخذتها من بين لحييها فقالرسول الله (ص): ما كان ينبغى لك أن تنعقيها اى تأخذى بعنقها و تعصريها

[33] Ibid., p. 318:

أهديت الى النبى (ص) لقحة فأمرنى أن أحلبها فحلبتها فجهدت حلبها؛ فقال (ص): لا تفعل! دع داعى اللبن.

Ma'āni al-Akhbār, p. 284, cited in *Bihār al-Anwār*, vol. 64, p. 149, no. 1; *Usd al-Ghābah,* vol. 3, p. 39:

أن رجلا حلب عند النبى (ص) ناقةً، فقال النبيُّ (ص): دع داعى اللبن.

[34] Kulayni, *Al-Furu' min al-Kāfi*, vol. 6, p. 212, no. 2 and 3; *Wasā'il al-Shi'ah,* vol. 16, pp. 239-40, Chapter 28, no. 1 and 2:

عن أبى عبدالله (ع) قال: قال رسول الله (ص): لا تأتوا الفراخَ فى أعشائها و لا الطير فى منامها حتى يصبح. فقال له رجلٌ: ما منامه يا رسول الله؟

قال (ص): الليل، منامه؛ فلا تطرقه فى منامه حتى يصبح؛ و لا

تأتوا الفراخ فى عُشّه حتى يريش و يطير؛ فاذا طار، فاوتر له
قوسك و انصب له فخّك. أيضاً أنه قال: نهى رسول الله (ص) عن
بيات (اتيان) الطير بالليل و قال: انّ الليلَ، أمانٌ لها

35 *Hayāt al-Haywān al-Kubrā*, Ibid, vol. 2, p. 208:

قال (ص): كان فيمن قبلكم، رجل يأتى وكر طائر؛ كلما أفرخ،
أخذ فراخه. فشكى ذالك الطائر الى الله تعالى ما يفعل به؛ فأوحى
الله تعالى اليه ان عاد، فسأهلكه

36 *Hayāt al-Haywān al-Kubrā*, Ibid, vol. 1, pp. 191-92, cited in *Bihār al-Anwār*, vol. 64, pp. 71, 72 and 307:

ابن مسعود قال: كنا عند النبى (ص)، فدخل رجل غيضة فأخرج
منها بيضة حُمرة. فجاءت الحمرة تزفّ على رأس رسول الله و
اصحابه؛ فقال (ص) لأصحابه: أيّكم فجعَ هذه؟ فقال رجل: يا رسول
الله أخذت بيضها و فى رواية، أخذت فرخها فقال (ص): رُدّهُ!
رُدّهُ! رحمة لها

37 Ibid.

38 The Arabic text is as follows:

فى أوّل كتاب جنائز من حديث عامر الرام...قال بينما نحن عند
رسول الله (ص) اذا أقبل رجل عليه كساء و فى يده شىء قد لف
عليه طرف كسائه فقال: يا رسول الله انى لما رأيتك أقبلتك فمررت
بغيضة شجر فسمعت فيها أصوات فراخ طائر فأخذتهن فوضعتهن
فى كسائى؛ فجائت أمهن فاستدارت على رأسى فكشفت لها عنهن
فوقعت عليهن، فلففتها معهن و ها هن فيه معى؛ فقال رسول الله
(ص): ضعهن عنك، فوضعتهن و أبت أمهن الا لزومهن. فقال
النبى لأصحابه: أتعجبون لرحمة ام الفراخ فراخها؟ قالوا: نعم يا
رسول الله! قال (ص): فوالذى بعثنى بالحق نبياً، الله أرحم بعباده
من أم هؤلاء الافراخ بفراخها! ارجع بهن حتى تضعهن من حيث
أخذتهن؛ فرجع بهن و أمهن ترفرف عليهن.

39 *Man Lā Yahduruhu al-Faqih*, vol. 2, p. 187; *Al-Khisāl*, vol. 1, p. 160 , cited in *Bihār al-Anwār*, vol. 64, p. 201, no. 1 and 2 and p. 210, no. 16; *Al-Fusul al-Muhimmah*, vol. 3, p. 348, chapter 75, no. 3077; *Mizān al-Hikmah*, Ibid, vol. 3, p. 1344, no. 4524:

على بن ابى طالب (ع) قال: قال رسول الله (ص) للدابّة على
صاحبها، خصال ستّ: يبدء بعلفها اذا نزل؛ و يعرض عليها الماء
اذا مر به؛ و لا يضرب وجهها، فانها تسبح بحمد ربها؛ و لايقف

على ظهرها الا فى سبيل الله عز و جل؛ و لا يحملها فوق الطاقة؛
و لا يكلّفها من المشى الا ما تطيق

[40] *Bihār al-Anwār*, vol. 64, p. 217 the last paragraph:

أنس بن مالك قال أن النبىّ (ص) قال: ...ثم قال: يجب على مالك
الدواب، علفها و سقيها لحرمة الرّوح

[41] *Man Lā Yahduruhu al-Faqih*, vol. 2, pp. 185-86; *Makārim al-Akhlāq*, p. 138, cited in *Bihār al-Anwār*, vol. 64, p. 159, no. 1 and p. 173, no. 24; *Thawāb al-A'māl*, p. 103, cited in *Bihār al-Anwār*, vol. 64, p. 167, no. 11 and p. 176, no. 36. Also refer to Ibid, p. 168, no. 14 and 17 and p. 175, no. 32. Also refer to: *Hayāt al-Haywān al-Kubrā*, vol. 2, p. 218; *Usd al-Ghābah*, vol. 2, p. 364 and vol. 5, p. 326:

قال رسول الله (ص): الخيل معقود بنواصيها الخير الى يوم
القيامة والمنفق عليها فى السبيل الله كالباسط يده بالصدقة لا
يقبضها....

[42] This mane also works as an awning for their necks in summer.

[43] *Makārim al-Akhlāq*, p. 138, cited in *Bihār al-Anwār*, vol. 64, p. 173, no. 25; *Usd al-Ghābah*, vol. 3, pp. 352 and 363:

روى عن رسول الله (ص) أنه قال: لا تجزّوا (لا تقصوا) نواصى
الخيل و لا أعرافها و لا أذنابها؛ فان الخير فى نواصيها و ان
أعرافها دفوءها و أذنابها، مِذابّها

[44] *Nawādir* by Rawandi, p. 34, cited in *Bihār al-Anwār*, vol. 64, p. 174, no. 29.

[45] *Majālis* by Ibn al-Shaykh, p. 244, cited in *Bihār al-Anwār*, vol. 64, p. 165, no. 9.

[46] *Hayāt al-Haywān al-Kubrā*, Ibid, vol. 2, p. 211; cited in *Bihār al-Anwār*, vol. 64, p. 177:

و روى أن تميما الدارىّ كان ينقّى شعيراً لفرسه و هو أمير على
بيت المقدس فقيل له: لو كلّفت هذا غيرك؟ فقال: سمعت رسولَ الله
(ص) يقول من نقّى شعيراً لفرسه ثم قام به حتى يعلفَه عليه، كتب
الله له بكلّ شعيرة حسنة عن مالك بن أنس انه قال: رباط يوم فى
سبيل الله خير من عبادة الرجل فى أهله ثلاثمائة و ستّين يوماً، كل
يوم ألف سنة

[47] Kulayni, *Al-Kāfī*, vol. 6, p. 539 cited in *Bihār al-Anwār* vol. 64, p. 214, no. 23:

أبى عبدالله (ع) قال: قال رسول الله (ص): لا تتورّكوا على الدواب
و لا تتّخذوا ظهورها مجالس

[48] *Kanz al-'Ummāl*, vol. 9, p. 63, no. 24957; *Mizān al-Hikmah*, vol. 3, p. 1344, no. 4519:

عنه (ص): اركبوا هذه الدواب سالمةً و ائدِعُوها سالمةً و لا
تتّخذوها كَراسِيَّ لأحاديثكم فى الطريق و الأسواق؛ فرب مركوبَة
خير من راكبها و أكثرَ ذِكُراللهِ تباركَ و تعالى منه

[49] *Bihār al-Anwār*, vol. 64, pp. 219 and 220; *Kanz al-'Ummāl*, vol. 9, p. 64, no. 24961:

أن النبيّ (ص) قال: أياكم أن تتّخذوا ظهور دوابّكم منابر؛ فان الله
تعالى انما سخّرها لكم لتبلغكم الى بلد لم تكونوا بالغيه الا بشقّ
الأنفس؛ و جعل لكم فى الأرض مستقرّاً فاقضوا عليها حاجاتكم

[50] *Kanz al-'Ummāl*, vol. 9, p. 62, no. 24951 and p. 67, no. 24980:

قال (ص): اتّقوا اللهَ فى هذهِ البهائمِ المعجمةِ؛ فاركبوها صالحةً و
كلوها صالحةً؛ و ايضاً قال (ص): اتّقوا اللهَ فى هذه البهائم؛ كلوها
سِماناً و اركبوها صالحةً

[51] Ibid., vol. 9, p. 62, no. 24952.

[52] Ibid., vol. 9, p. 69, no. 24992.

[53] *Bihār al-Anwār,* vol. 64, p. 219:

روى الطبرانى عن جابر رض أن النبيّ (ص) نهى أن يركب
ثلاثة على الدابّة

[54] *'Ilal al-Sharā'i'*, p. 194; *Al-Khisāl*, vol. 1, p. 49, cited in *Bihār al-Anwār*, Ibid, vol. 64, p. 203, no 4; *Kanz al-'Ummāl*, vol. 9, p. 66, no. 24971; *Mizān al-Hikmah*, vol. 3, p. 1344, no. 4523.

[55] *Man Lā Yahduruhu al-Faqih*, vol. 2, p. 191, cited in *Bihār al-Anwār*, vol. 64, p. 215, no. 25; *Kanz al-'Ummāl*, vol. 9, p. 62, no. 24950.

[56] *Al-Nihāyah*, vol. 5, p. 166; *Kanz al-'Ummāl*, vol. 9, p. 63, no. 24956.

[57] *Man Lā Yahduruhu al-Faqih,* vol. 2, p. 189, cited in *Bihār al-Anwār*, vol. 64, p. 213, no 21; *Mizān al-Hikmah*, vol. 3, p. 1344, no. 4518.

[58] Ibid..

[59] *Kanz al-'Ummāl*, Ibid, vol. 9, p. 66, no. 24973; *Mizān al-Hikmah*, vol. 3, p. 1344, no. 4520.

[60] *Kanz al-'Ummāl*, Ibid, vol. 9, p. 67, no. 24983.

[61] *Hayāt al-Haywān al-Kubrā*, vol. 2, p. 371:

أن النبى (ص) نهى عن تحريش بين البهائم و التحريش الاغراء و
تهييج بعضها على بعض كما يفعل بين الكباش و الديوك و غيرها

[62] *Hayāt al-Haywān al-Kubrā*, vol. 2, p. 371.

[63] *Bihār al-Anwār*, vol. 64, p. 277 and vol. 76, p. 331; *Kanz al-'Ummāl*, Ibid, vol. 9, p. 66, no. 24979 and p. 68, no. 24986-24989:

نهى رسول الله (ص) عن الوسم فى وجوه البهائم

[64] *Majālis al-Saduq*, p. 255; *Man Lā Yahduruhu al-Faqih*, vol. 4, p. 5, cited in *Bihār al-Anwār*, vol. 64, p. 215, no. 28 and p. 227, no. 19:

جعفر بن محمد عن آبائه (ع) قال: نهى النبىّ (ص) عن ضرب
وجوه البهائم و نهى عن قتل النحل و نهى عن الوسم فى وجوه
البهائم

Bihār al-Anwār, vol. 64, p. 217:

عن ابى سعيد خدرى أن النبىّ (ص) قال: لا تضربوا وجوه
الدواب، فان كل شىء يسبّح بحمده

Tafsir al-'Ayyāshi, cited in *Bihār al-Anwār*, vol. 64, p. 228, no. 25:

عن جعفر بن محمد عن أبيه (ص) قال: نهى النبىّ (ص) عن
توسم البهائم فى وجوهها و أن يضرب وجوه البهائم؛ فأنّها تسبّح
بحمد ربّها

Nawādir by Ravandi, pp. 14 and 15, cited in *Bihār al-Anwār*, vol. 64, p. 210:

قال على (ع): نهى رسول الله (ص) أن توسم الدواب، فرب دابّة
مركوبة خير من راكبها و أطوع لله تعالى و أكثر ذكراً

Al-Kāfi, vol. 6, p. 538, cited in *Mizān al-Hikmah*, vol. 3, p. 1346, no. 4528:

قال (ص): لا تضربوا الدوابّ فأنّها تسبّح بحمد الله.

[65] *Usd al-Ghābah*, vol. 2, p. 31.

[66] *Al-Tabaqāt al-Kubrā*, vol. 7, pp. 48 and 184.

Aspects of Environmental Ethics: An Islamic Perspective

Mohammad Ali Shomali

> Prophet Muhammad: *If Resurrection is starting, and one of you has a sapling in his hand which he can plant before he stands up, he must do so.*[1]

> Imam Sadiq (d. 148/765): *There is no joy in life unless three things are available: clean fresh air, abundant pure water, and fertile land.*[2]

One of the most important problems in today's world is the environmental crisis. It seems that this problem started when modern man stopped understanding himself as the vicegerent and trustee of the All-Merciful God who must channel divine mercy to everything at his disposal or within his reach, and stopped understanding nature as a sacred sign and valuable trust from God. For the same reason, it seems that the best way to protect the environment from destruction and, indeed, to improve its condition is to revive these forgotten understandings by referring back to the teachings and instructions of divine religions and reviewing and readjusting our policies regarding the application of modern technology and in using natural resources appropriately. In this paper, I will try to briefly present some aspects of the Islamic perspective on environmental ethics in the light of Qur'anic verses and Islamic narrations (hadiths). The paper consists of four parts: (I) nature, (II) governing rules in Islamic environmental ethics, (III) virtues related to human treatment of the environment, and (IV) vices related to human treatment of the environment.

I. Nature

Nature in general: There are more than 750 verses in the Qur'an that are related to nature. Fourteen chapters of the Qur'an are named after certain animals and natural incidents, such as: "the Cow," "the Cattle," "the Thunder," "the Bee," "the Ant," "the Daybreak," "the Sun," "the Night," "the Fig" and "the Elephant." Moreover, there are many cases in which God takes an oath by some natural phenomena like: "the dawn" (89:1) and "the fig and olive" (95:1). In numerous verses, the Qur'an states that all the natural phenomena have awareness of God and glorify God:

> And We made the mountains and the birds to celebrate our praise along with David. (21:79; 38:18)

> And there is not a thing but that it glorifies Him with His praise but you do not understand their glorification. (17:44)[3]

In many verses, the natural phenomena are characterised as divine signs indicating the knowledge, the wisdom and the power of God, such as:

> Most surely in the creation of the heavens and the earth and the alternation of the night and the day, and the ships that run in the sea with that which profits men and the water that God sends down from the cloud, then gives life with it to the earth after its death and spreads in it all (kinds of) animals, and the changing of the winds and the

clouds that are made subservient between the heaven and the earth, there are signs for a people who understand. (2:164)[4]

Water

In Islamic culture, water is very highly regarded. The word *"mā'"* (water) is used in the Qur'an about 60 times. Water is introduced as the origin and the source of life. For example, the Qur'an says: "And We have made of water everything living" (21:30).[5] The Qur'an (24:45) also states that God created from water every animal that goes on its belly, on two legs and on four legs, of water. Water is pure and purifying (25:48). Imam Sadiq said: "Surely God made the earth pure as He made the water pure."[6] A Muslim who wants to perform ritual prayer or to touch the Holy Qur'an or to circumambulate around the Ka'bah in Mecca must be ritually pure and to be ritually pure he needs to make ritual ablution with water. In Islamic symbolism, water normally stands for knowledge and faith or even for Imams. According to some traditions, the expression "the abundant water" in verse (72:16) esoterically refers to_abundant knowledge and faith and the expression "the flowing water" in verse (67:30) to Imam Mahdi.

Water must be kept pure and clean. For example, Imam Baqir (a) is quoted as saying: "Do not urinate in water!"[7]

Earth

Every Muslim in his ritual prayer has to prostrate to God several times on the earth (or an earthly material like soil or sands). If water is not available or using water is harmful to one's health (e.g. because of injury), one needs to use earth or earthly materials in a special way to perform ritual ablution.

In Islamic scriptures, the earth is introduced as an origin for the creation of human beings.

The Qur'an says:

From it (earth) We created you and into it We shall send you back and from it We will raise you a second time. (20:55)

Likewise, the earth is introduced as "a mother" for human beings. The Holy Prophet is quoted as saying:

Preserve the earth because it is your **mother**.[8]

God created the earth and laid it out for humanity.[9] He also made the earth manageable and tractable.[10] God has made for people a means of their livelihood in the earth.[11] Human beings should utilise the earth and construct upon it. The Holy Qur'an says: "He is the one who created you from the earth and settled you upon it, so that you might cultivate the land and construct towns and cities in which to live." (11:61) Imam Ali (a) says: "God has sent Adam to make the earth flourish by the help of his offspring."[12] Imam Ali (a) in a letter to his governor said: "You should be more concerned with the construction (physical development) of the land than collecting the land tax."[13] Elsewhere, he said: "Fear God regarding His servants and lands! You are responsible for the lands and the animals."[14]

Plants

Islam highly recommends planting trees and urges people to protect them to the extent that planting a tree is considered as an act of worship, for which special prayer is recommended. The Holy Prophet said: "Unless you are compelled, do not cut down a tree!"[15] Before battles, the Prophet always gave instruction to his soldiers not to harm women, children, the elderly, and those who surrendered and not to destroy or burn farms and gardens.[16]

In addition to the protection of plants, there are many hadiths that recommend Muslims to plant and farm. For example, the Prophet (s) said:

Whoever plants a tree and then a human or a creature of God eats its fruit, it will be considered as an act of charity for him.[17]

Whoever waters a date or lote tree it is as if he has given a drink to a thirsty believer.[18]

Imam Sadiq (a) said:

Farm and plant! By God, there is no occupation more lawful and pleasant than this.[19]

The best occupation is farming.[20]

The greatest alchemy is farming.[21]

Animals

According to Islamic teachings, animals have numerous rights, for which human beings are held responsible. In addition to the above-mentioned hadith from Imam Ali, peace be upon him (in which he says, "You are responsible for the lands and the animals"), one may refer to a hadith from Imam Sadiq (a): "There are six rights for the beasts that their owners should observe: they should not be forced to carry what they do not have the strength to bear, they should not be ridden while the rider is speaking, they should be given their provisions when they stop, they should not be branded (imprinted) or burnt, they must not be stricken at their face because they glorify God and they should be allowed to drink when they pass by water.[22] Imam Ali (a) condemned urinating in the water because there are animate creatures in it.[23]

A fundamental right for animals is the right to life. According to a well-known hadith, the Holy Prophet (s) said: "A woman will be put in the hell because she imprisoned a cat until the cat died."[24] The Prophet also said: "Whoever kills a sparrow without any reason will be questioned by God on the Day of Judgment."[25] Hunting birds or animals for fun is prohibited.[26] A very

165

outstanding scholar, 'Allamah Mohammad Taqi Ja'fari concludes his discussion about animals in this way:

> Consideration of whole sources of Islamic jurisprudence (*fiqh*) leads to the conclusion that animals must not be killed unless there is a legal permission (by God) like benefiting from them or being safe from their harm. There are adequate reasons for prohibiting hunting animals for fun and one can argue from these reasons for prohibition of killing animals without having a permitting cause.[27]

According to Islamic hadiths, an animal's life not only must not be taken unjustifiably, but also their life must be protected. The great Shi'a jurist, Zayn al-Din al-'Amili, known the Second Martyr (*al-Shahid al-Thāni*), in his *Masālik al-Afhām* writes:

> In the same way that spending money for saving a human being is compulsory, spending money to save a respected animal is compulsory, even if that animal belongs to another person.[28]

Elsewhere he stresses the necessity of buying medicine for animals when they become ill.[29] One of the greatest contemporary Shi'a jurists, Mohammad Hasan al-Najafi, writes:

> If by using water for making ritual ablution one is worried that an animal whose life is respected may become thirsty he must make *tayammum* (that is, ablution with soil instead of water), even though that animal is a dog.[30]

Elsewhere he declares that amongst animal rights is the right for a house, a place for rest. He says:

> It is compulsory to provide animals with what they need like food, water and a place.[31]

Animals must also be loved and respected. It is reported that Imam Ali (a) said: "Whoever curses an animal, he himself will be cursed by God."[32] An animal like a sheep or camel must not be slaughtered in front of another one.[33]

II. Governing rules in Islamic environmental ethics

Some of the major instructions on how to treat the environment and natural resources can be formulated as follows:

II.I. Benefit from natural resources in a responsible way!

Emphasis of the Qur'an and hadiths on nature and natural phenomena does not imply that we cannot benefit from them. Indeed, the Qur'an clearly suggests that God has created them in a way that man can dominate and benefit from them. For example, the Qur'an says:

> And the earth, He has set it for people. (55:10)

> He it is who created for you all that is in the earth.
> (2:29; 45:13; 31: 20; 16:10-14; 22: 65; 14:32-34)

The benefits that we take from the environment are not limited to material or physical ones. They also include mental and psychological benefits as well:

> And He created the cattle for you, you have in
> them warm clothing and many (uses) advantages,
> and of them you can eat. And there is beauty in
> them for you when you drive them back home and
> when you send them forth to pasture. (16:5 and 6)

There are some Qur'anic verses and Islamic hadiths which state the spiritual or psychological benefits of plants:

> And send down for you water from the cloud; then
> we cause to grow thereby beautiful and delightful
> gardens. (27:60; 50:7; 22:5)

167

The Holy Prophet (s) said:

> There are three things which cause brightness of
> the eyes: to look at greenery, running water and a
> beautiful face.[34]

As said before, nature and natural phenomena are also signs of
God, on which we should reflect to come to a better
understanding of God and a closer relationship with Him. We
also need some of the natural materials for performance of some
acts of worship. Therefore, we can benefit from them
theologically and spiritually as well.

II.II. Behave towards nature as a guardian!

Not only must man use natural resources in a responsible way,
but also, as the vicegerent of God on the earth (2:30; 6:165;
35:39), he must feel responsible for their maintenance and
improvement of their condition. The Holy Qur'an says:

> He is the one who created you from the earth and
> settled you upon it so that you might cultivate it
> and construct towns. (11.61)

Failure to observe divine pleasure and carry out his
responsibilities towards himself and the world certainly leads to
man's dissatisfaction as well as the destruction of the world. To
make the case theologically clearer, I can briefly say that God is
the Truth and the entire creation is based on the Truth. Following
the Truth leads to tranquillity of the heart and ultimate
satisfaction as well as an abundance of divine blessings including
both material and spiritual ones. For example, the Holy Qur'an
says:

> And if the people of the towns had believed and
> guarded (against evil) We would certainly have
> opened up for them blessings from the heaven and

the earth, but they rejected, so we overtook them for what they had earned. (7:96)

On the other hand, arrogance and selfishness before the Truth leads to confusion, forgetting one's self, the breakdown of human relations and even severe damage to the physical world. This is against the laws of the creation and, as a result, the world would resist such people and finally would rebel and save itself from ultimate corruption. This may be one way of understanding the following verse:

> And should the truth follow their low (carnal) desires surely the heavens and the earth and all those who are therein would have perished and been corrupted. (23:71)

II.III. Recognize your role as a trustee!

The Holy Qur'an states: "We offered the trust unto the heavens and the earth and the hills but they shrank from bearing it and were afraid of it. And man assumed it" (33:72).This means that human beings have been given the responsibility of stewardship and trust (al-amānah) by God in order to care for and serve as a channel for the blessings of God to all creation. Humans are invested with a special status and responsibility as trustees on earth and must fulfil the requirements of that trust.[35] According to Islamic thought, nature is a divine trust and man is the trustee. It can also be argued that since future generations also have rights in respect to nature with which to benefit, nature is also a trust for them.

II.IV. Plan for the improvement of your life and the whole world!

It is possible that religious people who believe in the eternal life and its superiority over the material life may underestimate the worldly life and its affairs. They may think that this is a transient state which expires very quickly and therefore they should

169

concentrate only upon the spiritual life and the Hereafter. It is true that the eternal life is to occupy the central place in our attention and actions. However, Islam teaches that we must do our best for the improvement and development of this world as well. For example, Imam Hasan (a) is quoted as saying: "In respect to your worldly affairs, act as if you are going to live here forever, and in respect to your afterlife, act as if you are going to die tomorrow!"[36] This hadith indicates that we need to be fully prepared for our eternal journey and must have the greatest possible provision for that, because there is a realistic possibility that we may die tomorrow and we may not have any further opportunities. Moreover, for our eternal journey, we need so many provisions that even if we work hard day by day, it will still be insufficient, even if we are given, so to speak, a very long life. On the other hand, we must work hard for this world as if we are going to live here forever. But a very important point is that this is not a realistic possibility; no one is going to remain in this world. This shows maximum emphasis because people may tend to undervalue working for the improvement of this world when they know that they live here temporarily. To overcome this problem they are asked to suppose that they would live in this world forever. Moreover, the hadith suggests that you must not only be concerned with yourselves and your immediate children. You must suppose that there will be a kind of continuity for your presence in this world through your offspring and through your fellow human beings. I should like to finish this section with a hadith from the Holy Prophet (s):

> There are six things that will be beneficial for a believer even after his death: a child who asks God's forgiveness for him, a book that remains from him, a tree that he plants, a well that he digs, a charity which he gives, and a good conduct that he establishes and is practiced by others after him.[37]

III. Some virtues related to human treatment of the environment

III.I. Cleanliness

Tidiness and cleanliness is very important in Islam. In respect to cleanliness, the Prophet (s) said: "Surely God is clean and loves the clean, so clean your courtyard."[38] He also said: "Be as clean as you can."[39] He also said: "Cleanliness is next to godliness."[40] He also said: "Surely Islam is clean, so be clean, because nobody can enter Paradise except he who is clean."[41] The Prophet told his wife: "Surely the clothes glorify, (but) when they are dirty and unclean they do not glorify."[42] Imam Ali (a) said: "Tidy (clean) clothes eliminate grief and sorrow."[43] These hadiths show that cleanliness has effects on the soul as well.

III.II. Moderation and balance

A believer should be moderate in all aspects of his life including his use of nature. The Holy Prophet (s) said: "The best of affairs is the medium one."[44] He also said: "Whoever is moderate he will not become poor."[45] Indeed, the whole world is based on order and harmony (mizān).[46] Exceeding limits in using nature or natural resources is extravagance which is considered as a major sin in Islam. For example, the Qur'an says:

> And eat and drink and be not extravagant, surely He does not love the extravagant (7: 31)

> And do not squander wastefully. Surely the squanderers are friends of satans and Satan is ever ungrateful to his Lord (17: 26- 27).

III.III. Thankfulness

Another important quality of a believer is thankfulness, not only in words, but also by deeds. Thankfulness by deeds means to use divine blessings in the way which is right and, therefore, pleasing to God. To misuse divine blessings or harm them for example by destroying jungles and polluting water are signs of ungratefulness which is severely condemned in Islam. For example, the Qur'an says: "Have you not seen those who have changed God's favour for ungratefulness and made their people to alight in the abode of perdition?" (14:28)

IV. Some vices related to the human treatment of the environment

IV.I. Extravagance

One of the great threats for human society and the environment is extravagance. The origins of this are greed and negligence. This character is controlled by religious teachings. In Islamic sources, two sins are distinguished. One is *isrāf* or wasteful consumption. Another sin is *tabdhir* or squandering. These two concepts are brought into play to adjust human behaviour.[47]

IV.II. Vandalism

According to a well-established rule in Shi'ite jurisprudence, nobody can cause harm or loss to others. This is a general rule which is supported by many verses and hadiths and, in particular, by the well-known prophetic hadith: *"La darara wa la dirara fi'l-Islam."* This hadith, about which tens of books and essays have been written, means that there is no place in Islam for inflicting any harm on one's self or on others.

IV.III. Corruption

Islam opposes mischief and corruption in all forms. Any act of mischief is condemned, whether it be in respect to human beings or living beings or even non-living beings. The Holy Qur'an says:

> When he turns his back, his aim is to spread mischief on the earth and destroy crops and progeny. But God does not love corruption. (2:205)

Do no mischief on the earth, after it has been set in order, but call on Him with fear and longing (in your hearts): for the Mercy of God is near to those who do good. (7: 56) [48]

Conclusion

In this paper, I have tried to address some aspects of environmental ethics from an Islamic perspective. We saw that great emphasis has been put in the Qur'an on nature and natural phenomena as divine signs indicating the knowledge, the wisdom and the power of God. Then we focused on four major parts of the environment, i.e., water, earth, plants and animals. In Islamic scriptures, water is introduced as the origin and the source of life and the earth is introduced as an origin for the creation of human beings and as our "mother." In Islam, planting trees is considered as an act of worship, for which special prayer is recommended and people are urged to protect them. Animals have numerous rights, including the right to life, the right to food and water, the right to shelter and the right for medicine. An animal's life can only be taken with the permission of God. Not only must an animals' life not be taken unjustifiably, but their life must also be protected. Animals must also be loved and respected.

Thus, it becomes clear that in Islam the environment is sacred and has an intrinsic value. Even if there is no threat or shortage, we still must look after natural resources, protect animals and plants and, more generally, improve and develop the environment. As the vicegerents of God, we have to channel the mercy of God to everything within our reach.

Bibliography

Radi, Sayyid Muhammad ibn Musa, *Nahj al-Balāghah* (Beirut: Dār al-Uswah, 1415 A.H.).

'Amili, Zayn al-Din, *Masālik al-Afhām* (various editions).

Najafi, Mohammad Hasan, *Jawāhir al-Kalām* (Beirut: Dār Ihyā' al-Turāth al-'Arabai).

Majidi, Ghulam Husayn ed. (1379), *Nahj al-Fasāhah* (Qum: Ansariyan, 1379 S.A.H.).

Kulayni, Mohammad, *Usul al-Kāfi* (Tehran: Dar al-Kutub al-Islamiyyah, 1397 A.H.).

Reyshahri, Mohammad, *Mizan al-Hikmah* (Qum: Dār al-Hadith, various editions).

Hurr al-'Amili, Mohammad, *Wasā'il al-Shi'ah* (Qum: Ismā'iliyan, 1392 A.H.).

Majlesi, Mohammad Baqir, *Bihār al-Anwār* (Beirut: Al-Wafā, 1983).

Ja'fari, Mohammad Taqi, *Rasā'il Fiqhi* (Tehran: Mu'assise-ye 'Allamah Ja'fari, 2002)

---

[1] *Nahj al-Fasahah,* vol. 2, p. 713.

[2] *Bihār al-Anwār*, vol. 75, p. 234.

[3] See also verses 13:13, 17:44, 24:41, 59:1, 61:1, 57:1, 59:24, 64:1 and 62:1.

[4] See also verses 3:191-192, 6:97, 6:99, 14:32-34, 16:10-16, 31:31, 35:12 and 13, 42:32-35, 45:3-6, 51:20 and 55:19-25.

[5] See also verses 56:68-70 and 22:5.

[6] Hurr al-'Amili, *Wasā'il al-Shi'ah,* vol. 1, p. 133.

[7] Ibid., pp. 240 and 241.

[8] *Nahj al-Fasāhah*, no. 1130.

[9] See e.g. verse 55:10.

[10] Verse 67:15 says: "It is He Who has made the earth manageable for you..."

[11] Verse 7:10 says: "God has given you (mankind) power on earth and appointed therein a livelihood for you."

[12] *Nahj al-Balāghah.*

[13] Ibid., Letter No. 53.

[14] Ibid., Sermon 167. Also cited in *Bihār al-Anwār*, vol. 32, p. 9.

[15] *Wasā'il al-Shi'a*, vol. 11, pp. 43 and 44.

[16] See e.g. *Al-Kāfi*, vol. 5, pp. 29 and 30.

[17] *Nahj al-Fasahah*, vol. 2, p. 563.

[18] Hurr al-Amili, *Wasā'il al-Shi'a*, vol. 17, p. 42.

[19] *Al-Kāfi*, vol. 5, p. 260.

[20] Ibid.

[21] Ibid.

[22] *Al-Kāfi*, vol. 6, p. 537.

[23] *Wasā'il al-Shi'ah*, vol. 1, p. 240.

[24] Nahj al-Fasahah, no. 1559.

[25] *Nahj al-Fasahah*, no. 2224 and no. 2610.

[26] See e.g. *Wasā'il al-Shi'a*, vol. 8, p.481.

[27] *Rasā'il-e Fiqhi*, p. 250. Elsewhere he writes: "Hunting animals for amusement and without need is prohibited. Therefore, if someone makes a trip for such kind of hunting his trip is a sinful trip." (Ibid., p. 118)

[28] *Masālik al-Afhām*, vol. 2, p. 250.

[29] Ibid., vol. 1, p. 305.

[30] *Jawāhir al-Kalām*, vol. 5, p. 114.

[31] Ibid., vol. 31, p. 395.

[32] *Wasā'il al-Shi'ah*, vol. 8, p. 356.

[33] Ibid., vol. 16, p. 258.

[34] *Nahj al-Fasāhah*, no. 1291 & *Bihār al-Anwār*, vol. 3, p.129.

[35] For example, see verses (23:8) and (4: 58).

[36] Hurr al-'Amili, *Wasā'il al-Shi'a,* vol. 17, p. 28.

[37] Ibid., vol. 2, p. 44.

[38] *Nahj al-Fasāhah,* no. 703.

[39] Ibid., no. 1182.

[40] Ibid., no. 3161.

[41] Ibid., no. 612.

[42] *Mizān al-Hikmah,* vol. 10, no. 3898.

[43] *Wasā'il al-Shi'ah,* vol. 3, p. 346.

[44] *Nahj al-Fasāhah,* no. 1481.

[45] Ibid., no. 2509.

[46] For the significance of the concept of *mizān,* see commentaries of the Qur'an on the verse 55:7-9.

[47] See also III.II.

[48] See also the verses 7:85; 13:25; 16:88; 26:152; 27:48; 47:22.